ACHILLES TENDON
CURRENT CONCEPTS

Second Edition

DJO PUBLICATIONS

A DJO Global, Inc. initiative
International Headquarters - London

www.DJOpublications.com

Project Assistant: Maayke N. van Sterkenburg
Project Manager: Francine Van Steenkiste
Book and Cover Design: Lee Millington
Illustrations: Gemma Hatherley
Production: Matthew Blackwell
Compositor: DJO Publications (DJO Global, Inc.)

First edition 2008
Second edition 2008

ISBN number: 978-0-9558873-0-7

Published by DJO Publications
1a Guildford Business Park
Guildford
Surrey
GU2 8XG
UK
www.DJOglobal.eu

Printed in the UK

ACHILLES TENDON RUPTURE

CURRENT CONCEPTS

Second Edition

EDITORS:

C. Niek van Dijk
MD, PhD
Professor and Chief of Service
Department of Orthopaedic Surgery and Traumatology
Academic Medical Centre/ University of Amsterdam
Amsterdam, the Netherlands

Jon Karlsson
MD, PhD
Professor of Orthopaedics and Sports Traumatology
Department of Orthopaedics
Sahlgrenska University Hospital
Sahlgrenska Academy at Göteborg University
Göteborg, Sweden

Nicola Maffulli
MD, MA, PhD, FRCS
Professor of Trauma and Orthopaedic Surgery
Keele University
Stoke-on-Trent, UK

Hajo Thermann
MD, PhD
Centre for Knee and Foot Surgery
Atos-Clinic Centre
Heidelberg, Germany

LIST OF CONTRIBUTORS

Paul W. Ackermann
MD, PhD
Orthopaedic Laboratory
Department of Molecular Medicine
and Surgery
Karolinska Institutet
Stockholm, Sweden

Per Aspenberg
MD, PhD
Section for Orthopaedics
Institute for Neuroscience and
Locomotion
Faculty of Health Sciences, Linköping
University
Linköping, Sweden

Francesco Benazzo
MD
Clinic for Orthopaedics and Trauma
University of Pavia
Foundation IRCCS Policlinics San
Matteo

James D.F. Calder
MD, FRCS, FFSEM
Consultant Orthopaedic Surgeon
North Hampshire Hospitals
Foundation Trust
Basingstoke, UK
Clinical Senior Lecturer
Imperial College, London, UK

C. Niek van Dijk
MD, PhD
Professor and Chief of Service
Department of Orthopaedic Surgery
and Traumatology
Academic Medical Centre/ University
of Amsterdam
Amsterdam, the Netherlands

Brian G. Donley
MD
Director, Centre of Foot and Ankle
Surgery
Associate Professor of Surgery
Department of Orthopaedic Surgery
Cleveland, Ohio

Robin R. Elliot
MA, FRCS
Specialist Registrar Trauma and
Orthopaedics
Royal Bournemouth Hospital
Bournemouth, UK

Karin Grävare- Silbernagel
PhD
Physical Therapist
Lundberg Laboratory of Orthopaedic
Research
Department of Orthopaedics
Göteborg University, Sahlgrenska
University Hospital
Physical Therapy & Sports Medicine
Clinic
Göteborg, Sweden

Jon Karlsson
MD, PhD
Professor of Orthopaedics and Sports
Traumatology
Department of Orthopaedics
Sahlgrenska University Hospital
Sahlgrenska Academy at Göteborg
University
Göteborg, Sweden

Gino M.M.J. Kerkhoffs
MD, PhD
Orthopaedic Surgeon
Department of Orthopaedic Surgery
Academic Medical Centre
Amsterdam, the Netherlands

Karsten Knobloch
MD, PhD
Consultant for General Surgery
Plastic, Hand and Reconstructive
Surgery
Hannover Medical School
Hannover, Germany

Michael Lutz
FRACS
Foot and Ankle Fellow
North Hampshire Hospitals Founda-
tion Trust
Basingstoke, UK

Nicola Maffulli
MD, MA, PhD, FRCS
Professor of Trauma and Orthopaedic
Surgery
Keele University
Stoke-on-Trent, UK

Mario Mosconi
MD
Clinic for Orthopaedics and Trauma
University of Pavia
Fondazione IRCCS Policlinico San
Matteo

Stefano M.P. Rossi
MD
Clinic for Orthopaedics and Trauma
University of Pavia
Foundation IRCCS Policlinics San
Matteo

Murali K. Sayana
MBBS, MS, AFRCSI
Dept of Trauma and Orthopaedics
Royal College of Surgeons in Ireland
St. Stephens Green
Dublin, Ireland

Maayke N. van Sterkenburg
MD
PhD fellow
Orthopaedic Research Centre
Amsterdam
Department of Orthopaedic Surgery
Academic Medical Centre
Amsterdam, the Netherlands

Aimee C. Stroink
MD
Resident Orthopaedic Surgery
Department of General Surgery
Westfries Gasthuis
Hoorn, the Netherlands

Masato Takao
MD, PhD
Professor & Chief, Foot & Ankle Unit
Department of Sports Medicine
Department of Orthopaedic Surgery
Teikyo University School of Medicine
Tokyo, Japan

Hajo Thermann
MD, PhD
Centre for Knee and Foot Surgery
Atos-Clinic Centre
Heidelberg, Germany

Richard G.H. Wallace
MCh, MD, FRCS
Consultant Trauma and Orthopaedic
Surgeon
Musgrave Park Hospital
Belfast, Northern Ireland, UK

Giacomo Zanon
MD
Clinic for Orthopaedics and Trauma
University of Pavia
Foundation IRCCS Policlinico San
Matteo

CONTENTS

PREFACE

'The Achilles tendon, if bruised or cut, causes the most acute fevers, induces choking, deranges the mind, and at length brings death'. (Hippocrates)

Achilles tendon ruptures are relatively common. Although the Achilles tendon, formed by the merging of the tendons of gastrocnemius and soleus, is the thickest and strongest tendon in the human body, it remains susceptible to injury. During the last two decades, the incidence of spontaneous ruptures has been rising, probably because of the increasing keep-fit culture. Approximately 75% of Achilles tendon ruptures occur during sports activities. Several aetiological hypotheses have been proposed, including the adverse influence of corticosteroids, fluoroquinolone antibiotics, exercise- induced hyperthermia, and mechanical abnormalities of the foot. The diagnosis of an acute rupture can usually be made clinically. Recently, several meta-analyses on management were published, but there is still a lack of consensus on the best management of the acute Achilles tendon rupture. Management can be broadly classified into operative and non-operative treatment. Generally, open operative management has been used in athletes and young, fit patients, percutaneous operative in those who do not wish to have an open repair, and non-operative management in the elderly. Recent systematic reviews have concluded that operative management has a lower rerupture rate, but must be balanced by the risks associated with surgery. Recent studies have demonstrated the beneficial effect of functional aftertreatment in a mobile cast or brace.

The purpose of this book is to provide the reader with the latest information concerning aetiology, diagnosis, and management of acute ruptures of the Achilles tendon.

In 2007, the Achilles Tendon Study Group was founded to promote the research and scientific study of injuries to the Achilles tendon. The Study Group meets over one day every year. In the even years, the meeting takes place in the same venue of and immediately before the biannual ESSKA 2000 Congress. The other years, the meeting takes place in the same venue of and immediately before the biannual ISAKOS Congress.

This book on the management of acute ruptures of the Achilles tendon is the first product of the group, and is part of an upcoming current concepts series on ailments of the Achilles tendon. The best available evidence and expert opinion was collected and discussed in an international panel of expert orthopaedic surgeons. The outcome is collected in this book, of which the production was made possible by DJO. Having read this first issue, we hope that orthopaedic surgeons, trauma surgeons, and residents will find it a complete and comprehensive collection of current evidence on the aetiology, diagnosis and treatment of acute ruptures of the Achilles tendon.

The Editors

"As in ruptures of the Achilles tendon, its etiology is likely to be multifactorial."

(S.Young)

Chapter 1.

AETIOLOGY

Murali K. Sayana, Nicola Maffulli

Take Home Message

• *The aetiology of Achilles tendons rupture is multifactorial.*
• *Spontaneously ruptured Achilles tendons in healthy individuals often have degenerative changes histologically.*
• *After 30 years of age, there is sequential decrease in the maximum diameter and density of collagen fibrils of Achilles tendon. However, there is little evidence of failed healing response.*
• *Drugs like flouroquinolones and steroids may predispose to tendon ruptures.*
• *Hyperthermia within the relatively avascular Achilles tendon makes it more prone to rupture.*
• *Mechanical factors such as overpronation of the foot on heel-strike, training errors, malfunction or suppression of the proprioceptive component of skeletal muscle predispose to Achilles tendon rupture.*

Introduction

There is little agreement on the aetiology of spontaneous Achilles tendon ruptures. Inflammatory and autoimmune conditions, genetically inherited collagen abnormalities, infectious diseases, and neurological conditions have been implicated in the aetiology of a spontaneous rupture[2,14,15,32]. The blood flow in the tendon decreases with increasing age[19], and the site of the Achilles tendon typically prone to rupture is relatively avascular compared with the rest of the tendon[30,31,42]. A disease process may predispose the tendon to spontaneous rupture even when exposed to minor trauma[34].

Tendon degeneration and rupture

Histological evidence of collagen degeneration in all 74 ruptured Achilles tendons was reported by Arner and co-workers[2]. However, in that study nearly two-thirds of the specimens were obtained more than 48 hours after the rupture. Davidsson and Salo reported marked degenerative changes in two patients with a rupture of the Achilles tendon who had an operation on the day of the injury[13]. The changes, therefore, should be regarded as having developed before the rupture. Waterston and co-workers reported that specimens from all Achilles tendon ruptures that were operated on within twenty-four hours after the injury showed marked degenerative changes and collagen disruption, in accordance with the findings in another recent study[22,50]. Alternating exercise with inactivity could produce the changes seen in tendons[29]. Sports in addition to daily activities place additional stress on the Achilles tendon, leading to the accumulation of trauma, which, although below the threshold for frank rupture, could lead to secondary intratendinous degenerative changes[16,50].

The aging tendon

Strocchi and co-workers studied the age related morphometric changes in human Achilles tendon[46]. They reported decrease in the average, maximum diameter and density of collagen fibrils and an increase of fibril concentration with increasing age. Sargon and co-workers studied Achilles tendon biopsies under transmission electron microscope in ultra thin specimens obtained from 28 subjects with an age range between 1 and 68 years (4 subjects per each decade)[41]. The transverse diameters of collagen fibres were measured. The specimens from 1-9 years age group, 10-19 years and 20-29 years showed increasing trend with means of 69.8 nm, 96.1 mm and 222 nm respectively. However, there was a decreasing trend in the later groups, 30-39 years, 40-49 years, 50-59 years; > 60 years had a mean diameter of 159 nm, 148 nm, 76.4 nm and 68.7 nm respectively. They postulated that the decrease observed in the diameters of collagen fibres of 30 - 45 year-old patients, who are in an active period of their life, can play a role in the aetiology of the frequency of Achilles tendon ruptures in this age group. These specimens were obtained from patients undergoing Achilloplasty for contracture or from ruptured tendons. Therefore, the study could have had the drawback of examining ruptured or degenerated tendons in 30-60 years age group and subjects with Achilles tendon contracture in the 1-29 years age group who did not have healthy normal tendons. However, it is likely that collagen fibrils in the normal healthy tendons may undergo a similar change with aging. Jozsa and co-workers reported that intact human Achilles tendons consisted of fibrils with a diameter of 30 - 80 nm[23]. In contrast, ruptured and degenerated human tendons displayed 2 distinct populations of fibrils of 40 - 60 and 10 - 20 nm. In our own studies[50], the Achilles tendons of aged individuals with no history of tendon ailments showed no evidence of tendinopathy, with no histological appearance of failed healing response or degeneration.

Corticosteroids and Rupture of the Tendon

Intralesional and perilesional corticosteroids are administered for a variety of diseases and have been widely implicated in tendon ruptures. Injection of hydrocortisone into the calcaneal tendons of rabbits caused necrosis at the site of injection 45 minutes after the injection, and these tendons showed a delayed healing response compared with those that had received an injection of saline solution[3]. The anti-inflammatory and analgesic properties of corticosteroids may mask the symptoms of tendon damage, inducing individuals to maintain high levels of activity even when the tendon is damaged[8]. Corticosteroids interfere with the healing cascade, which depends on inflammation, and intratendinous injection of corticosteroids results in weakening of the tendon for up to 14 days[25]. The disruption is directly related to collagen necrosis, and restoration of the strength of the tendon is attributable to the formation of an acellular amorphous mass of collagen. Therefore, vigorous activity should be avoided for at least fourteen days after a corticosteroid injection in the vicinity of a tendon[25]. Unverferth and Olix reported a rupture in five athletes who had been given injections of corticosteroids in the region of the Achilles tendon for the management of tendinopathy[48]. Residua of the corticosteroids were found at the site of the rupture in four of the five patients. A meta-analysis recently has shown that corticosteroid injections do not seem to play a beneficial role in the treatment of Achilles tendinopathy[45]. Orally administered corticosteroids also have been implicated in the aetiology of tendon rupture. Over a 10 year period, 12 patients with a rupture of the Achilles tendon had been on long-term oral corticosteroid therapy for the treatment of chronic obstructive small airways disease in our centre. Four of them sustained a bilateral injury[37]. Some studies have not demonstrated deleterious effects of corticosteroids, and therefore some argue that it still is not possible to pinpoint the aetiological role of these agents[33]. For example, McWhorter and co-workers demonstrated that a single injection of hydrocortisone acetate in a traumatized calcaneal tendon of a rat had no important biomechanical or histological adverse effect[35].

A recent retrospective safety study of low volume peri-tendinous steroid injections under fluoroscopic control for Achilles tendinopathy had reported only 1 minor complication in 43 patients, who had a minimum of 2-year follow up[17]. Koenig and co-workers reported improvement of pain and improvement in colour Doppler following ultrasound-guided intratendinous glucocorticoid injection into tendopathic tendons in five patients[28]. However, given the present evidence, prolonged oral administration and repeated peritendinous and intratendinous injection of corticosteroids should be avoided.

Fluoroquinolones and Rupture of the Tendon

Pefloxacin, ofloxacin, levofloxacin, norfloxacin and ciprofloxacin are the fluoro-quinolones most often associated with tendon disorders. Nalidixic acid, a qui-nolone is not as toxic to the tendons as the fluorinated quinolones. Extremely few cases of tendon toxicity have been reported for nalidixic acid to the WHO database over the years. In contrast to fluoroquinolones, nalidixic acid does not alter the mitochondrial activity in tenocytes[4]. There is laboratory evidence of di-rect deleterious effects of fluoroquinolones on tenocytes.

Pefloxacin, does not affect transcription of type-I collagen but decreases the transcription of decorin at a concentration of only 10-4 millimoles [4]. The result-ing decrease of decorin may modify the architecture of the tendon, altering its biomechanical properties, and produce increased fragility.

Ultrastructural changes in the Achilles tendon of rats treated with fluoroquinolo-nes showed typical findings consist of multiple vacuoles and large vesicles in the cytoplasm of tenocytes due to swellings of mitochondria and endoplasmic retic-ulum, densified nuclei and clumped chromatin[43,44]. Furthermore, there is a gen-eral decrease in the fibril diameter and an increase in the distance between the fibrils. These changes are dose-dependent and persist for a considerable time[43]. Animals receiving fluoroquinolone in doses close to those administered to hu-mans showed disruption of the extracellular cartilage matrix, which exhibited the development of fissures and chondrocyte necrosis, and depletion of collagen[47]. The abnormalities seen in animals might also occur in humans. Szarfman and co-workers recommended that the labelling on packaging for fluoroquinolone be updated to include a warning about the possibility of tendon rupture. In its recommendations on the use of this class of antibiotics, the British National For-mulary suggested that "at the first sign of pain or inflammation, patients should discontinue the treatment and rest the affected limb until the tendon symptoms have resolved"[9].

In France, between 1985 and 1992, 100 patients who were being managed with fluoroquinolones had tendon disorders, which included 31 ruptures[40]. Many of these patients also had received corticosteroids, which means that it is difficult to implicate only the fluoroquinolones. Surveillance studies suggested that levo-floxacin related tendon rupture occurred in less than 4 per million prescriptions according to American data[24]. Prescription of fluoroquinolones for benign infec-tions or to elderly patients with corticosteroid treatment should be avoided, and, for any fluoroquinolone prescription, the risk/benefit ratio should be carefully considered[36].

Hyperthermia and Rupture of the Tendon

Up to 10% of the elastic energy stored in tendons may be released as heat[26]. Wil-son and Goodship evaluated the temperatures generated in vivo within equine superficial digital flexor tendons during exercise[51]. A peak temperature of 45°C, a temperature at which tenocytes can be damaged[1], was measured within the core of the tendon after just seven minutes of trotting. Exercise-induced hyperthermia therefore may contribute to tendon degeneration. Abundant blood supply to tissues should help to cool overheating. However, the Achilles tendon, which has relatively avascular areas, may be more susceptible to the effects of hyperthermia.

The Mechanical Theory

McMaster proposed that a healthy tendon would not rupture, even when subjected to severe strain[34]. However, Barfred demonstrated that, if straight traction were applied to a tendon, as in McMaster's experiments, the risk of rupture would be distributed equally to all parts of the muscle-tendon-bone complex[7,8,9]. If oblique traction was applied, the risk of rupture would be concentrated on the tendon. He calculated that, if a 1.5-centimeter-wide Achilles tendon in a human were subjected to traction with 30° of supination on the calcaneus, the fibres on the convex aspect of the tendon would be elongated by 10% before the fibres on the concave side would be strained. Therefore, the risk of rupture would be greatest when the tendon was obliquely loaded, when the muscle was in maximum contraction, and when the initial length of the tendon was short. Such factors are probably all present in movements occurring in many sports that require rapid push-off. Barfred's theory is largely supported by that of Guillet and co-workers (reported in a study by Postacchini and Puddu[38]), who proposed a purely traumatic theory for rupture of the tendon in young healthy patients.

A healthy tendon may rupture after a violent muscular strain in the presence of certain functional and anatomical conditions. These include incomplete synergism of agonist muscle contractions, a discrepancy in the thickness quotient between muscle and tendon, and inefficient action of the plantaris muscle acting as a tensor of the Achilles tendon. Participation in sports plays a major role in the development of problems with the Achilles tendon, and training errors are a major factor[10,18,20,38]. The flared heel on most sport shoes forces the hindfoot into pronation when the heel strikes the ground, and the heel tabs on some shoes may play a similar role. Clement and co-workers, in a study on the aetiology of Achilles tendinopathy, found that 61 (56%) of 109 athletes displayed a so-called functional overpronation of the foot on heel-strike, with a whipping action of the Achilles tendon[11]. Exaggeration of this whipping action may lead to intratendinous microtears. Poor flexibility of the Gastrocnemius/soleus unit was also considered to contribute to overpronation[10,13]. Unequal tensile forces on different parts of the tendon may produce a so-called torsional ischemic effect, i.e. transient vasoconstriction of the intratendinous vessels, and therefore contribute to the vascular impairment already present within the Achilles tendon[11]. Inglis and Sculco proposed that malfunction or suppression of the proprioceptive component of skeletal muscle predisposes athletes to rupture of the Achilles tendon. They believed that athletes who resume training after a period of rest are particularly susceptible to rupture of the Achilles tendon as a result of this malfunction[21].

X-ray diffraction spectra were used to study the behaviour of the structure of collagen during tendon-loading by Knörzer and co-workers[27]. Healthy tendons without previous degenerative changes are damaged initially at the submicroscopic fibrillar level. The process of intrafibrillar sliding occurs a few seconds before macroscopic slippage of collagen fibres. Accumulation of fibrillar damage, therefore, results in rupture of tendons unaffected by degenerative changes. Such findings support the theory that a complete rupture is the consequence of multiple microruptures, and that tendon damage must reach a critical point, after which failure occurs.

Fourteen weeks of strength training increased patella tendon stiffness and Young's modulus, in older humans. As a consequence, tendon elongation and strain were reduced, decreasing the possibility of tendon strain injury in old age. Similarly, strength training for gastrocnemius may help reduce the strain on the Achilles tendon and thereby rupture[39].

References

1] Arancia G, Crateri Trovalusci, P, Mariutti G, Mondovi B. Ultrastructural changes induced by hyperthermia in Chinese hamster V79 fibroblasts. Internat J Hyperthermia 1989;5:341-350.

2] Arner O, Lindholm Å, Orell SR. Histologic changes in subcutaneous rupture of the Achilles tendon. A study of 74 cases. Acta Chir Scandinavica 1958-1959,116: 484-490.

3] Balasubramaniam P, Prathap K. The effect of injection of hydrocortisone into rabbit calcaneal tendons. J. Bone and Joint Surg 1972;54-B:729-734.

4] Bernhard-Beaubois K, Hecquet C, Hayem G, Rat P, Adolphe M: In vitro study of cytotoxicity of quinolones on rabbit tenocytes. Cell Biol Toxicol 1998;14:283-292.

5] Barfred T. Kinesiological comments on subcutaneous ruptures of the Achilles tendon. Acta Orthop Scandinavica 1971;42:397-405.

6] Barfred T. Experimental rupture of the Achilles tendon. Comparison of experimental ruptures in rats of different ages and living under different conditions. Acta Orthop Scandinavica 1971;42:406-428.

7] Barfred T. Experimental rupture of the Achilles tendon. Comparison of various types of experimental rupture in rats. Acta Orthop Scandinavica 1971;42:528-543.

8] Beskin JL, Sanders RA, Hunter SC, Hughston JC. Surgical repair of Achilles tendon ruptures. Am J Sports Med 1987;15:1-8.

9] British National Formulary. London, British Medical Association, Royal Pharmaceutical Society of Great Britain, 1996;32:259.

10] Clain MR, Baxter DE. Achilles tendinitis. Foot and Ankle 1992;13:482-487.

11] Clement DB, Taunton JE, Smart GW. Achilles tendinitis and peritendinitis: etiology and treatment. Am J Sports Med 1984;12:179-184.

12] Davidsson L, Salo M. Pathogenesis of subcutaneous tendon ruptures. Acta Chir Scandinavica 1969;135:209-212.

13] Davidson RG, Taunton JE. Achilles tendinitis. Med Sports Sci 1987;23:71-79.

14] Dent CM, Graham GP. Osteogenesis imperfecta and Achilles tendon rupture. Injury 1991;22: 239-240.

15] Dodds WN, Burry HC. The relationship between Achilles tendon rupture and serum uric acid level. Injury 1984;16:94-95.

16] Fox JM, Blazina ME, Jobe FW, Kerlan RK, Carter VS, Shields CL Jr, Carlson GJ. Degeneration and rupture of the Achilles tendon. Clin Orthop 1975;107:221-224.

17] Gill SS, Gelbke MK, Mattson SL, Anderson MW, Hurwitz SR. Fluoroscopically guided low-volume peritendinous corticosteroid injection for Achilles tendinopathy. A safety study. J Bone and Joint Surg;86-A:802-6.

18] Gross MT. Chronic tendinitis: pathomechanics of injury, factors affecting the healing response, and treatment. J Orthop and Sports Phys Ther 1992;16:248-261.

19] Håstad K, Larsson LG, Lindholm Å. Clearance of radiosodium after local deposit in the Achilles tendon. Acta Chir Scandinavica 1958-1959;116:251-255.

20] Hess GP, Cappiello WL, Poole RM, Hunter SC. Prevention and treatment of overuse tendon injuries. Sports Med 1989;8:371-384.

21] Inglis AE, Sculco TP. Surgical repair of ruptures of the tendo Achillis. Clin Orthop 1981;156:160-169.

22] Jarvinen M, Józsa L, Kannus P, Jarvinen TL, Kvist M, Leadbetter W. Histopathological findings in chronic tendon disorders. Scandinavian J Med and Sci Sports 1997;7:86-95.

23] Jozsa L, Reffy A, Balint JB. Polarization and electron microscopic studies on the collagen of intact and ruptured human tendons. Acta Histochem 1984;74:209-215.

24] Kahn JB. Latest industry information on the safety profile of levofloxacin in the US. Chemotherapy 2001;47(Suppl. 3):32-37.

25] Kennedy JC, Willis RB. The effects of local steroid injections on tendons: a biomechanical and microscopic correlative study. Am J Sports Med 1976; 4:11-21.

26] Ker RF. Dynamic tensile properties of the plantaris tendon of sheep (ovis aries). J Exper Biol 1981;93:283-302.

27] Knörzer E, Folkhard W, Geercken W, Boschert C, Koch MH, Hilbert B, Krahl H, Mosler E, Nemet-schek-Gansler H, Nemetschek T. New aspects of the etiology of tendon rupture. An analysis of time-resolved dynamic-mechanical measurements using synchrotron radiation. Arch Orthop and Trauma Surg 1986; 105:113-120.

28] Koenig MJ, Torp-Pedersen S, Qvistgaard E, Terslev L, Bliddal H. Preliminary results of colour Dop-pler-guided intratendinous glucocorticoid injection for Achilles tendonitis in five patients. Scand J Med Sci Sports;14:100-6.

29] Kristensen JK, Andersen PT. Rupture of the Achilles tendon: a series and a review of literature. J Trauma 1972;12:794-798.

30] Kuwada GT. Diagnosis and treatment of Achilles tendon rupture. Clin Podiat Med and Surg 1995;12:633-652.

31] Lagergren C, Lindholm Å. Vascular distribution in the Achilles tendon. An angiographic and micro-angiographic study. Acta Chir Scandinavica 1958-1959;116: 491-496.

32] Maffulli N, Irwin AS, Kenward MG, Smith F, Porter RW. Achilles tendon rupture and sciatica: a pos-sible correlation. British J Sports Med 1998;32:174-177.

33] Mahler F, Fritschy D. Partial and complete ruptures of the Achilles tendon and local corticosteroid injections. British J Sports Med 1992;26:7-14.

34] McMaster PE. Tendon and muscle ruptures. Clinical and experimental studies on the causes and location of subcutaneous ruptures. J Bone and Joint Surg 1933; 15:705-722.

35] McWhorter J.W, Francis RS, Heckmann RA. Influence of local steroid injections on traumatized tendon properties. A biomechanical and histological study. Am J Sports Med 1991;19:435-439.

36] Melhus A. Fluoroquinolones and tendon disorders. Expert Opin Drug Saf 2005;4:299.

37] Newnham DM, Douglas JG, Legge JS, Friend JA. Achilles tendon rupture: an underrated complica-tion of corticosteroid treatment. Thorax 1991;46: 853-854.

38] Postacchini F and Puddu G. Subcutaneous rupture of the Achilles tendon. Internat Surg 1976;61:14-18.

39] Reeves ND, Maganaris CN, Narici MV. Effect of strength training on human patella tendon me-chanical properties of older individuals. J Physiol 2003;1:548:971-981.

40] Royer RJ, Pierfitte C, Netter P. Features of tendon disorders with fluoroquinolones. Therapie 1994;49:75-76.

41] Sargon MF, Ozlu K, Oken F. Age-related changes in human tendo calcaneus collagen fibrils. Saudi Med J 2005;26:425-8.

42] Schmidt-Rohlfing B, Graf J, Schneider U, Niethard FU. The blood supply of the Achilles tendon. Internat Orthop 1992;16:29-31.

43] Shakibaei M, Pfister K, Schwabe R, Vormann J, Stahlmann R. Ultrastructure of Achilles tendons of rats treated with ofloxacin and fed a normal or magnesium-deficient diet. Antimicrob Agents Chem-other 2000;44:261-266.

44] Shakibaei M, Stahlmann R. Ultrastructural changes induced by the des-F(6)-quinolone garenoxacin (BMS-284756) and two fluoroquinolones in Achilles tendon from immature rats. Arch Toxicol 2003;77:521-526.

45] Shrier I, Matheson GO, Kohl HW. Achilles tendonitis: are corticosteroid injections useful or harm-ful? Clin J Sport Med 1996;6:245-250.

46] Strocchi R, De Pasquale V, Guizzardi S, Govoni P, Facchini A, Raspanti M, et al. Human Achilles ten-don: morphological and morphometric variations as a function of age. Foot Ankle 1991;12:100-104.

47] Szarfman A, Chen M, Blum MD. More on fluoroquinolone antibiotics and tendon rupture [letter]. New England J Med 1995;332:193.

48] Unverferth LJ, Olix ML. The effect of local steroid injections on tendon. In Proceedings of the

American Academy of Orthopaedic Surgeons. J Bone and Joint Surg 1973;55-A:1315.
49] Waterston SW. Histochemistry and biochemistry of Achilles tendon ruptures. B Med Sc dissertation, University of Aberdeen, Aberdeen, Scotland, 1997.
50] Waterston SW, Maffulli N, Ewen SW. Subcutaneous rupture of the Achilles tendon: basic science and some aspects of clinical practice. British J Sports Med 1997;31:285-298.
51] Wilson AM, Goodship AE. Exercise-induced hyperthermia as a possible mechanism for tendon degeneration. J Biomech 1994;27:899-905.

"Achilles absent, was Achilles still"

(Homer)

Chapter 2.

EPIDEMIOLOGY

Mario Mosconi, Giacomo Zanon, Stefano M.P. Rossi,
Francesco Benazzo

Take Home Message

• *Achilles tendon rupture incidence increased significantly in the last decades mainly in sports with abrupt repetitive jumping and sprinting movements.*
• *Men are significantly more involved than women, although incidence in women is increasing.*
• *There are two peaks of incidence: the first is sports activity-related, and occurs between 30 and 50 years of age. The second occurs after the age of 50 in non-athletes and women.*
• *Acute Achilles tendon ruptures are more frequent in elderly athletes, but caution should be taken in rehabilitation in younger athletes as rerupture is more frequent.*
• *Racial differences appear to exert a significant effect in Achilles tendon rupture, with ruptures being more frequent in Negroids.*

Introduction

In the last few decades the role of sports and physical activity has become more and more important in all modern societies. The risk of tendon injury has increased, and prevention is important.

Several studies indicate that participation in specific sports is associated with an increased risk of tendon injury[15,19], but cohort-based studies on long-term cumulative incidence are lacking.

The lifetime cumulative incidence of Achilles tendinopathy among former endurance runners was higher than previously reported at 52%[10]. Long-term consequences of tendon problems for today's athletes after their sport career were larger than previously anticipated[10].

In a cross-sectional study of 214 athletes and non-athletes between the ages of 17-66, ultrasonographic measurements of the Achilles tendon were performed on all participants[9]. Overall, patients who were active athletes sought medical care more often than those who did not participate regularly in sports. Twenty-seven (33%) young athletes had Achilles tendon pathology, compared with 9 (14%) younger non-athletes. A total of 36 (64%) elderly athletes were diagnosed with Achilles tendon disorders, compared with 15 (26%) elderly people who were not sports active. Moreover, in this study, microtears, acute tendinopathy and peritendinopathy were associated with younger age. Calcifications and partial or complete rupture were mainly seen in the elderly subjects.

The exact incidence of the different types of Achilles tendinopathies is difficult to ascertain because of the high number of clinical entities, the absence of uniformity in the classifications used by the different authors, and because different clinical scenarios may co-exist (e.g., insertional tendinopathy with peritenditis, etc.).

Incidence of Achilles tendon ruptures

Physical activity

The best data available for Achilles tendon ruptures come from studies on badminton players. In 66 elite players in Sweden 21 of 66 players (32%) have had a disabling painful condition of the Achilles tendon during the last 5 years, while 17% had an ongoing problem. In 12 of 21 players (57%), the condition involved the midportion of the tendon[4]. In a middle-aged group of badminton players, 44% complained of Achilles tendon problems, and a positive correlation was found only between symptoms and age[5].

In another study, 95 of 1405 recruits (6.8%) suffered from Achilles tendinopathy (in 94%, it was a peritendinopathy) with a significant difference between winter (9.4%) and summer (3.6%)[16].

The prevalence of Achilles tendinopathy in runners is estimated to be approximately 6% - 11%, and 16% of a running population were forced to give up indefinitely.

As far as the ruptures are concerned, an increase of Achilles tendon ruptures during the last decades has been noted.

Josza and co-workers reported the Achilles tendon to be the most frequently ruptured tendon, accounting for 40% of all tendon ruptured requiring surgery[8].

Gender and age

Most Achilles tendon ruptures occur in men, with a ratio from 2:1 to 18:1[2,13]. Leppilahti and co-workers showed an increasing incidence of rupture from 2/100000 inhabitants in 1979-1986 to 7/100000 in 1987-1994[12]. The incidence of ruptures in Scotland increased from 4.7/100.000 in 1981 to 6/100.000 in 1996, more in females than males[14], even if men outnumber women by 7:1.

The incidence of Achilles tendon ruptures in the city of Edmonton between 1998 and 2002 ranged from an annual average of 5.5 to 9.9 ruptures per 100000 inhabitants, with an overall mean of 8.3/100000 subjects[20]. There was a significant difference in Achilles tendon ruptures over the last two study years for both genders (women, $p<0.02$; men, $p<0.03$). The mean age for patients with an Achilles tendon rupture was 40.6 years for men and 44.5 years for women. Achilles tendon ruptures occurred most frequently in the 30-39 and 40-49 year old age groups in both men and women.

In a Danish study[6], the annual incidence of Achilles tendon ruptures increased from 18.2/100000 in 1984 to 37.3/100000 in 1996. The peak of incidence in sports-related injuries occurred in the 30-49 age group, while the peak of incidence in ruptures not related to sports occurred in older patients (50-59 years group).

Achilles tendon ruptures are often associated with sports involving repetitive jumping and sprinting. Housian and co-workers showed that more than 70% of ruptures occurred in sporting activities as badminton, soccer and handball[6]. In a study by Inglis, basketball players were most frequently injured[7], while for Cretnik soccer players[2] were. Houshian and co-workers showed that 74.2% of the ruptures were sports-related, and 89% of these occurred in ball and racket games[6].

The incidence of rerupture is approximately 4-5%[12,18]. Rettig and co-workers suggested that Achilles tendon ruptures in a younger population (<30 years) have a higher rerupture rate than similar injuries in an older age group (31-50 years), in which the injury is more common. They conclude that early weight-bearing and an early range of motion rehabilitation protocols, although favourable in the elder athlete, should be avoided in the younger ones, although this blanket statement is controversial in the light of recent trends[18].

The risk of contralateral tendon rupture is significantly increased in patients who suffered an Achilles tendon rupture. Årøen and co-workers reported an overall incidence of Achilles tendon rupture of 8/100000 per year in a population of 320000 inhabitants. 10/168 (6%) experienced an acute rupture of the contralateral Achilles tendon in the follow-up period (4.2 years), an incidence of 1410/100000 per year in this selected population[1].

Race

People from Negroid origin appear to be more prone to this type of injury when compared to Caucasian or Asian populations, even if the racial difference in tendon ruptures are not well studied.

Davis and co-workers suggested that there may be predisposing factor(s) that result in a higher risk of Achilles tendon ruptures in Negroid individuals[3].

More recently, based on the hypothesis that race is a risk factor for major tendon ruptures, White and co-workers identified 52 major tendon ruptures in a study of patients admitted for surgical management in a hospital of North Carolina. The rate of major tendon rupture was 13 times greater for Negroid people in this study population when compared with Caucasians[21].

In a recent study, Owens and co-workers estimate the rate of major tendon rupture per 1000 person-years, while controlling for differences in gender, service, rank, and age for quadriceps, patellar and Achilles tendon ruptures[17]. It appears that there is a significant relative predisposition towards lower-extremity major tendon rupture in Negroid U. S. service members when compared with Caucasian service members.

Davis and co-workers studied 865 military recruits, who underwent Achilles tendon surgical repair in 1994-1996 in a US Military hospital showing that Negroids were at increased risk of undergoing repair of the Achilles tendon compared with Caucasians and suggesting that besides Negroids having a significantly increased risk for injury related to playing basketball than Caucasians and Asians, there may be other predisposing factor(s) that result in a higher risk of Achilles tendon ruptures in Negroid individuals[3]. Further investigations on racial risk factor are needed.

References

1] Arøen A, Helgø D, Granlund OG, Bahr R. Contralateral tendon rupture risk is increased in individuals with a previous Achilles tendon rupture. Scand J Med Sci Sports 2004;14:30-33.

2] Cretnik A, Frank A. Incidence and outcome of rupture of the Achilles tendon. Wien Klin Wochenschr 2004;116, Suppl 2:33-38.

3] Davis JJ, Mason KT, Clark DA. Achilles tendon ruptures stratified by age, race, and cause of injury among active duty U.S. Military members. Mil Med 1999;164:872-873.

4] Fahlström M, Lorentzon R, Alfredson H. Painful conditions in the Achilles tendon region: a common problem in middle-aged competitive badminton players. Knee Surg Sports Traumatol Arthrosc 2002;10:57-60.

5] Fahlström M, Lorentzon R, Alfredson H. Painful conditions in the Achilles tendon region in elite badminton players. Am J Sports Med 2002;30:51-54.

6] Houshian S, Tscherning T, Riegels-Nielsen P. The epidemiology of Achilles tendon rupture in a Danish county. Injury 1998;29:651-654.

7] Inglis AE, Sculco TP. Surgical repair of ruptures of the tendo Achillis. Clin Orthop Relat Res 1981;156:160-169.

8] Josza L, Kvist M, Balint BJ, Reffy A, Jarvinen M, Lehto M, Barzo M The role of recreational sport activity in Achilles tendon rupture. A clinical, pathoanatomical, and sociological study of 292 cases. Am J Sports Med 1989;17:338-343.

9] Krolo I, Visković K, Ikić D, Klarić-Custović R, Marotti M, Cicvara T.
The risk of sports activities--the injuries of the Achilles tendon in sportsmen. Coll Antropol 2007;31:275-278.

10] Kujala UM, Sarna S, Kaprio J. Cumulative incidence of Achilles tendon rupture and tendinopathy in male former elite athletes. Clin J Sport Med 2005;15:133-135.

11] Leppilahti J, Puranen J, Orava S. Incidence of Achilles tendon rupture.
Acta Orthop Scand 1996;67:277-279.

12] Leppilahti J, Forsman K, Puranen J, Orava S. Outcome and Prognostic Factors of Achilles Rupture Repair Using a New Scoring Method. Clin Orthop Relat Res 1998;346:152-161.

13] Levi N. The incidence of Achilles tendon rupture in Copenhagen. Injury 1997;28:311-313.

14] Maffulli N, Waterston SW, Squair J, Reaper J, Douglas AS.
Changing incidence of Achilles tendon rupture in Scotland: a 15-year study. Clin J Sports Med 1999;9:157-160.

15] Maffulli N, Wong J, Almekinders LC. Types and epidemiology of tendinopathy. Clin Sports Med 2003;22:675-692.

16] Milgrom C, Finestone A, Zin D, Mandel D, Novack V.
Cold weather training: a risk factor for Achilles paratendinitis among recruits. Foot Ankle Int

2003;24:398-401.

17] Owens B, Mountcastle S, White D. Racial differences in tendon rupture incidence. Int J Sports Med 2007;28:617-620.

18] Rettig AC, Liotta FJ, Klootwyk TE, Porter DA, Mieling P. Potential risk of rerupture in primary Achilles tendon repair in athletes younger than 30 years of age. Am J Sports Med 2005;33:119-123.

19] Schepsis AA, Jones H, Haas AL: Achilles tendon disorders in athletes. Am J Sports Med 2002;30:287-305.

20] Suchak AA, Bostick G, Reid D, Blitz S, Jomha N. The incidence of Achilles tendon ruptures in Edmonton, Canada. Foot Ankle Int 2005;26:932-936.

21] White DW, Wenke JC, Mosely DS, Mountcastle SB, Basamania CJ. Incidence of major tendon ruptures and Anterior Cruciate Ligament tears in US Army soldiers. Am J Sport Med 2007;35:1308-1314.

> *"The repair of an injured Achilles tendon can be enhanced by time-dependent application of inflammatory mediators and mechanical stimuli."*
>
> *(P. Ackermann)*

CHAPTER 3.

HEALING AND REPAIR MECHANISM

Paul W. Ackermann, James D.F. Calder, Per Aspenberg

Take Home Message

• *Achilles tendon repair is regulated by a complex temporal interaction of inflammatory mediators and neuromediators combined with graded mechanical stimuli.*
• *Achilles tendon repair, in animals, can be promoted by application of growth factors (e.g. CDMP, PDGF, TGF-β), thrombocyte concentrate, neuromediators (eg. SP) and external mechanical stimuli.*
• *Acceleration of Achilles tendon repair in patients is a clinically relevant issue, but requires meticulous testing of the above mentioned principles.*

Key players in tendon healing

Connective tissue repair and tendon healing is a highly dynamic process involving complex interactions of various blood and tissue derived cells, inflammatory mediators and extracellular matrix molecules. The immediate goal in repair is to achieve tissue integrity, homeostasis and load bearing capability.

In response to an injury, the wound site is directly infiltrated with blood derived cells (platelets, leukocytes, monocytes and lymphocytes, Table 1) initiating the inflammatory response by release of inflammatory mediators (Table 2). As a result of the inflammatory mediators tissue derived cells (macrophages, fibroblasts, myofibroblasts, endothelial cells, mast cells), (Table 3) are triggered to transform and activate production of extracellular matrix and collagen type III. Following cell activation, the healing tendon proper, which normally is practically devoid of nerves and vessel, is successively infiltrated by new nerves and vessels providing essential neuro-vascular mediators for the repair process[1,2,20].

BLOOD DERIVED CELLS

CELL	ACTION	MEDIATOR
Platelets	Wound hemostasis	PDGF, TGF-B, FGF, EGF, B-thromboglobulin, histamine, serotonin, bradykinin, prostaglandins, prostacyclin, and thromboxane. PF4, C5a complement, PAF, leukotriene B4
Neutrophils	Phagocytosis and wound debridement	Proteolytic enzymes
Monocytes	Monocytes transform into macrophages	IL-2, TNF-a, PDGF, and IFN-y stimulate transformation
Lymphocytes	Regulate tissue remodeling: Pro-inflammatory T cells Anti-inflammatory helper T cells	Pro-Inflammatory: IL-2, IFN-y, and TNF-B Anti-inflammatory: IL-4-6, IL-10, and IL-13

Table 1: Infiltration of wound site with blood derived cells in response

INFLAMMATORY MEDIATORS

GROUP	ACTION	MEDIATOR
Eicosanoids	Vasodilation Vasoconstriction Vascular permeability Chemotaxis	Prostaglandins: Vasodilation Prostacyclin: Vaso-,bronchodilation Thromboxanes: Vasoconstriction Leukotrienes: Vasoconstriction, increased vascular permeability Lipoxins: Chemotaxis
Cytokines	Act on hematopoietic cells to modulate immune or repair processes by controlling cellular growth, differentiation, metabolism, and protein synthesis	Chemokines: Proinflammatory, attract and activate leukocytes. Lymphokines: Produced by activated T lymphocytes Monokines: Produced by mononuclear phagocytes. Interleukins IL-1 – 23: Mainly IL-1 – 10 produced by macrophages, mast cells, and lymphocytes involved in healing.
Nitric Oxide	Vasodilation, vascular permeability, angiogenesis antimicrobial activity, antiplatelet aggregation activity. Collagen synthesis. Extracellular matrix	iNOS: vasodilation, antimicrobial activity, antiplatelet aggregation activity, and induction of vascular permeability. eNOS: angiogenesis, collagen synthesis

Growth Factors	Act on nonhematopoietic cells to modulate wound healing by stimulating protein production, extracellular matrix synthesis, matrix turnover, and cellular death	Epidermal growth factor ; EGF, TGF-α: Stimulates mesenchymal, epithelial, fibroblast and endothelial cell growth. Fibroblast growth factor; aFGF, bFGF: Stimulates angiogenesis, collagen synthesis, wound contraction, and proteoglycan synthesis. Insulin growth factor; IGF-I, IGF-II: Stimulates angiogenesis, and mitosis in fibroblasts and chondrocytes. Nerve growth factors; BDNF, NGF: Stimulates growth and differentiation of motor, sympathetic and sensory neurons. Platelet-derived growth factor; PDGF, VEGF: Chemotaxis and proliferation of eg. macrophages, fibroblasts, smooth muscle and endothelial cells. Transforming growth factor: TGF-β1, β2, β3: Macrophage and fibroblast chemotaxis, collagen synthesis, scar remodeling. BMPs 1-7, CDMPs 1-3: Induces bone, tendon, cartilage, and ligament tissue formation.

Table 2: Initiation of the inflammatory response by release of inflammatory mediators

Increasing mechanical load activates myofibroblasts and fibroblasts to increase the production of collagen type I to enlarge the callus size, and enhance the capacity to withstand high mechanical load. The ensuing succesive remodelling of the callus involves lymphocytes and mast cells which regulate matrix remodeling proteinases (MMPs) through release of cytokines. In combination with graded cellular load, a more organised internal arrangements is produced by, for example, improved cross-linking that leads into a smooth functional unit with enhanced mechanical tissue properties.

TISSUE DERIVED CELLS		
CELL	**ACTION**	**MEDIATOR**
Macrophages	Orchestrate healing by regulating angiogenesis, fibroplasia, and extracellular matrix synthesis. Wound débridement.	Fibroblast chemotaxis and proliferation: PDGF. Myofibroblast activation: TGF-B1, fibronectin. Other growth factors: EGF, IGF. Cytokines: TNF-a, IL-1,6, IFN-y. Débridement: Collagenase, elastase. Antimicrobial: NO, oxygen radicals
Fibroblasts	Collagen synthesis and myofibroblast transformation	PDGF released from macrophages stimulates proliferation of fibroblasts into the wound from the surrounding tissue
Myofibroblast	Type III collagen synthesis and contraction	The myofibroblast is derived from the fibroblast by macrophage release of TGF-B1 and adhesion to the extracellular matrix molecule, fibronectin
Endothelial Cells	Forming of capillary tubes by VEGF stimuli	Endothelial cells synthesize NO, which increases VEGF production
Mast Cells	Vascular permeability, tissue remodeling, neurotrophic	Vascular permeability: Histamine. Tissue remodeling: TGF-beta, IL-1 and IL-4, tryptase. Neurotrophic: NGF

Table 3: Tissue derived cells, triggered to transform and activate production of extracellular matrix and collagen type III

Temporal organisation of key players

Tendon healing occurs through both extrinsic and intrinsic mechanisms. The extrinsic theory considers the tendon as inert and avascular, with inflammatory response from and scar tissue formed by the surrounding tissues[21]. The intrinsic theory suggests that tendons are not inert, and can heal without an inflammatory response[17].

Achilles tendon healing occurs in three phases; inflammatory phase, a reparative collagen-forming phase, and a remodelling phase. Immediately after rupture, the defect is filled with blood clot and tissue debris and the inflammatory response begins. During the following 72 hours, granulation tissue is formed from the extrinsic peritendinous tissues and the intrinsic tissue of the epitenon and endotenon. This inflammatory phase continues for about 10 days, during which there is phagocytic removal of debris and minimal strength of repair from a fibrin clot.

During the first week, collagen synthesis commences and is maximal by week four – the reparative, collagen-forming phase. The glycoprotein, fibronectin, acts as a chemotactic agent for fibroblasts, which are the predominant cell type, and type III collagen is initially laid down perpendicular to the rupture. With loading of the tendon the orientation of the fibroblasts and collagen changes to the longitudinal axis of the tendon by 4 weeks post- injury[14].

By 4 weeks, the mechanical strength of the repair increases, as there is consolidation and remodelling of the maturing granulation tissue under tension, and the collagen synthesis changes from type III to type I[16].

Various factors influence the rate and strength of tendon healing. The most important is tension across the repair which speeds realignment of collagen fibres, increases tensile strength and minimises deformation at the repair site[15,27]. Early motion accelerates the nerve plasticity through regeneration and expression of neuromediator receptors)[5,6], and thereby possibly promotes the intrinsic mechanisms of repair from the epitenon, reducing the extrinsic response and subsequent ingrowth of tissues which may lead to adhesion formation. Gap formation at the repair site must be minimised, as this may lead to early re-rupture[26].

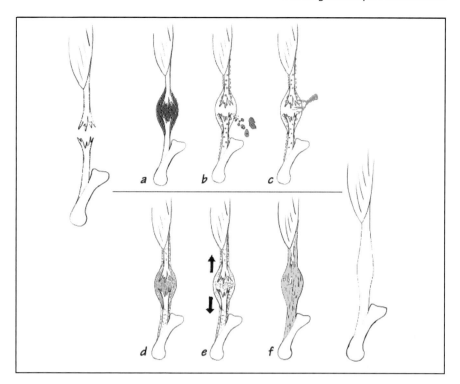

Figure 1: Scheme of tendon repair

a) Haematoma with infiltration of blood derived cells.
b) Invasion and transformation of tissue derived cells.
c) Vascular and neuronal ingrowth.
d) Loose collagenous callus formation.
e) Mechanical stimulation.
f) Maturation and remodelling.

Regulation of key players

It is possible to make injured tendons heal faster. Surprisingly little research has been perform to explore and exploit this possibility. Research on stimulation of tendon repair is still at the stage of animal experimentation. The by far most common experimental model for tendon repair uses the Achilles tendon of the rat.

Mechanical stimulation

Mechanical stimulation improves tendon repair, or rather, lack of mechanical stimulation is detrimental. Most animal models for evaluation of the effect of disuse on tendon apply external fixation, hind limb suspension, or surgical interventions such as denervation and disarticulation. A perhaps more specific model is to paralyze the gastrocnemius and soleus muscle complex with botulinum toxin to produce disuse without surgery or external fixation devices, as the botulinum toxin is specific for the acetylcholin signalling of the motor end plates. In rats with transected Achilles tendons, the botulinum toxin treatment had a drastic negative effect on tendon callus strength: two weeks after transection, force at failure was reduced to less than 30% of transected but loaded controls[27]. Rats in captivity have a sedentary life-style. If they are given an environment that stimulates to greater physical activity, the healing tendon callus becomes bigger and stronger[27]. Interestingly, increased activity also leads to shortening of the tendon callus, obviously via increased myofibroblastic activity, so that the separated tendon stumps come closer together (unpublished data).

A new way of applying mechanical stimulation to an immobilized tendon could be performed by using external intermittent pneumatic compression (IPC). IPC, which clinically is used to prevent thrombosis and increase blood circulation, has produced positive effects on wound and fracture healing, though the mechanisms are still largely unknown. Recently, however, IPC was demonstrated to enhance the neuro-vascular in-growth in a tendon repair model so as to increase the expression of sensory neuropeptides by up to 100%[8]. In the same model, IPC promoted tissue perfusion and accelerated both fibroblast proliferation and collagen organization during tendon repair[9]. Whether IPC can reverse the negative effects of immobilisation on tissue biomechanics still needs to be explored.

NSAIDs

The inflammatory phase of tendon repair seems to pave the way for the formation of a fibrous callus. If early inflammation is inhibited by, for instance, a cox inhibitor (NSAID) such as indomethacin, or a specific one, as valdecoxib, the fibrous callus can loose a third of its strength, due to inferior material properties[18]. This detrimental effect of early treatment survives the inflammatory phase, and can still be seen after 2 weeks in the rat[31]. If, on the other hand, NSAID treatment is started on the 6th day after injury, when the inflammatory phase is mostly over, there is instead a positive effect on the mechanical properties, so that we get/ resulting in a thinner tendon with better material properties and intact over-all strength (force at failure)[14,31].

Stimulation with GDFs (CDMPs)

Several growth factors stimulate tendon repair after exogenous protein application (Table 4). One of the problems with local application of growth factors is their short half-life and the associated need for a slow-release carrier, such as a collagen sponge[3] or a coated suture thread[22]. However, CDMPs can be injected in an acidic solution[10], because they are almost insoluble at neutral pH, and may precipitate when buffered by the tissue to neutral pH. A local injection of 10 micrograms of CDMP-1. –2, or –3 into the haematoma 6 hours after Achilles tendon transection leads to approximately 30% increase in total strength after 1 week in the rat[13]. In the rabbit, similar effects were seen at 2 weeks with 20 micrograms[12]. These two models used unsutured tendon defects allowing full weight-bearing. The patellar tendon in the rabbit can be unloaded by connecting the patella with the tibial tubercle with steel wires. A single injection of 20 µg CDMP into the haematoma after rabbit patellar tendon transection increased the strength of the repair by more than 65%[28], without an increase in callus transverse area. The increase in force at failure at mechanical testing arose entirely from improved

material properties.

Growth factor	Doses	Model	Evaluation	Time	Results	Reference
PDGF	0.5, 1 and 5 μg	Rat MCL	Mech	12 d	Dose-dependent benefical effect if administrated within 24 h.	Batten et al. 1996
PDGF-BB	400 ng, 20 μg.	Rabbit MCL	Mech, Hist	6 w	Improved ultimate load, energy and elongation	Hildebrand et al. 1998
PDGF-BB+TGF-beta-1	400 ng+4ng, 20 μg.+200 ng	Rabbit MCL	Mech, Hist	6 w	TGF-beta-1 did not lead to additional improvement	Hildebrand et al. 1998
FGF-2	0, 10, 100 and 1000 ng.	Rat patellar tendon, 1×4 mm window defect	Mech, IHC and pyridinoline crosslink analyses	7 and 14 d	Increased cell proliferation and type III collagen expession at 3 d	Chan et.al, 1997, 2000
VEGF	100 μl (50 μg/ml)	Rat AT repaired with suture	Mech	1, 2, and 4 w	Higher early tensile strength. Increased TGF-β expression	Zhang et al. 2003
IGF-1	25 μg	Rat AT transsection	Mech, functional	15 d	Reduced maximum functional deficit and accelerated recovery	Kurtz et al. 1999
TGF-beta-1	10 ng, 100 ng	Rats AT, transected and sutured	Mech, in situ hibridisation	1, 2, 4 w	A dose-depended increase in the expression of procollagen I and III mRNA. The failure load and stiffness increased by TGF-beta-1 at 2 and 4 weeks	Kashiwagi et al. 2004
BMP-7 (OP-1)	100 μg	Rats AT, transected, with or without denervation of the calf muscle or forefoot amputation	Mech, Hist	2 w	Reduced strength of tendon with or without mechanical unloading. Lots of bone	Forslund and Aspenberg, 1998
CDMP-1 CDMP-2	1 μg, 10 μg	Rats AT defect, denervation of the calf muscle	Mech, Hist	2 w	Tensile strength increased dose-dependently	Aspenberg and Forslund 1999
CDMP-1 (GDF-5 / BMP-12)	CDMP-1-coated suture	Rats AT transsected and sutured	Mech, Hist	1, 2, 4 and 8 w	Improved repair	Rickert et al. 2001
CDMP-2 (GDF-6 / BMP-13)	10 μg	Rabbits AT defect	Mech	8 d	CDMP-2 improved tendon repair. No bone or cartilage	Forslund and Aspenberg 2001
CDMP-1, 2 and 3	0, 0.4, 2 and 10 μg	Rats AT transsection	Mech, Hist	8 d, 4 w	Improved healing dose-dependently. Some bone and cartilage	Forslund et al. 2003
CDMP-2	0, 2, 10, or 50 μg	Rats AT defect	Mech	8 d	CDMP-2 improved tendon repair	Forslund and Aspenberg 2003

SP, NPY, VIP	75, 65, 100 pg	Rat MCL	Mech	2 w	SP, NPY, VIP all improved tendon repair	Grorud et al. 2006
SP	10(-6) μg	Rats AT transsected and sutured	Mech	1,2,6 w	SP improved stress and work at maximal load, but not stiffness.	Steyaert AE et al. 2006
NGF	10 μg	Rat MCL	Mech, Hist, blood flow	7, 14, 42 d	NGF increased failure load, ultimate tensile strength and stiffness at 42 d. Blood flow and reinnervation increased.	Mammoto et al. 2008

Table 4: Papers on applying growth factor protein to healing tendon or ligament

Platelet concentrate

Platelets contain a wide variety of growth factors, which are released at the site of injury. Several of these factors stimulate repair in various soft tissue models.
A single injection of a moderate amount of activated platelets into the haematoma 6 hours after tendon transection in the standard rat model increased force at failure after one week[4]. Moreover, the effect on tissue mechanics was largest as late as 3 weeks after transection. At this time, significantly better tissue organization could be demonstrated at histology[27].

How can it be possible that a single injection of thrombocytes can have effects on repair that lasts for several weeks? It seems counterintuitive, considering that the release of growth factors, and their survival, may be exhausted over some minutes to a few hours. If the healing tendon was unloaded with botulinum toxin, no stimulatory effect of a thrombocyte injection could be seen at 2 weeks. Thus, loading is required for a lasting effect. However, thrombocytes increased callus strength at 5 days, and the size of the callus at 3 days[27]. Thus, it seems that the thrombocyte injection caused a short-lived proliferative response. This early response produces a tissue which allows mechanical stimulation to begin earlier, leading to a better end result.

An important finding in the thrombocyte experiments was that the thrombin, which was used for activation the platelets, also has a small but significant stimulatory effect of its own. Indeed, thrombin can act as a growth factor. Continuous inhibition of thrombin activity decreases the size and strength of the tendon callus by approximately one third[30]. This is important, because it is being discussed whether patients with Achilles tendon ruptures should have routine prophylaxis against venous thrombosis. This prophylaxis acts through inhibition of thrombin (via factor Xa activity), and might have a negative effect on repair.

Neuronal factors

In addition to growth factors also neuromediators, so called neuropeptides that are released by ingrowing nerve fibres during tendon repair have essential effects on healing[1,2]. Thus, supplement of substance P in physiologic concentrations to healing Achilles tendons proved to enhance fibroblast aggregation and to increase tensile strength more than 100% compared with controls[7,24]. Another approach to increase nerve ingrowth and neuromediators presence at the injury site has been performed by administering nerve growth factor (NGF). In one study supplementation of NGF via osmotic pumps over 7 days after injury to healing medial collateral ligaments in rats promoted both reinnervation and angiogenesis resulting in enhanced mechanical properties[19].

Summary and clinical consideration

The goal of treatment in humans is to shorten immobilization, and indirectly through this produce a better functional end result. Another approach to counteract the detrimental effects of immobilisation might be to apply adjuvant external mechanical stimuli, for example by intermittent pneumatic compression. The mechanics of the healing human Achilles tendon has been measured 6 weeks after surgery via implanted markers, correlating strain with stress[23]. Variation between patients is very large. This appears to be the case also in other species with similar-sized Achilles tendons, such as sheep, where force at failure showed an unexplained variation, much larger that in rodents. The variation in humans suggests that there is room for improvement in at least some patients, but unfortunately it also means that clinical studies will have to be large to have a satisfactory statistical power.

In conclusion, Achilles tendon repair can be stimulated in animals, and methods for measuring tendon repair and function in humans have recently been developed.

References

1] Ackermann PW, Ahmed M, Kreicbergs A. Early nerve regeneration after Achilles tendon rupture – a prerequisite for healing? J Orthop Res 2002;20:849-856.

2] Ackermann PW, Li J, Lundeberg T, Kreicbergs A. Neuronal plasticity in relation to nociception and healing of rat achilles tendon. J Orthop Res 2003;21:432-441.

3] Aspenberg P and Forslund C. Enhanced tendon healing with GDF 5 and 6. Acta Orthop Scand 1999;70:51-54.

4] Aspenberg P, Virchenko O. Platelet concentrate injection improves Achilles tendon repair in rats. Acta Orthop Scand 2004;75:93-99.

5] Bring D K-I, Renström P, Ackermann PW. Physical activity modulates nerve plasticity and stimulates repair after achilles tendon rupture.
J Orthop Res 2007;25:164-172.

6] Bring D K-I, Reno C, Renström P, Salo P, Hart D, Ackermann PW. Joint Immobilization Reduces the Expression of Sensory Neuropeptide Receptors and Impairs Healing after Achilles Tendon Rupture in a Rat Model J Orthop Res, In press.

7] Burssens P, Steyaert A, Forsyth R, van Ovost EJ, Depaepe Y, Verdonk R. Exogenously administered substance P and neutral endopeptidase inhibitors stimulate fibroblast proliferation, angiogenesis and collagen organization during Achilles tendon healing. Foot Ankle Int 2005;26:832-839.

8] Dahl J, Li J, Bring D K-I, Renström P, Ackermann PW. Intermittent Pneumatic Compression enhances neuro-vascular ingrowth during connective tissue healing. A Study in the Rat. J Orthop Res 2007;25:1185-1192.

9] Dahl J, Li J, Fahlgren A, Aspenberg P, Bring D, Renström P, Ackermann PW. Intermittent Pneumatic Compression Enhances Healing in a Tendon Repair Transactions of the International Symposium on Ligaments and Tendons VII, 2007, San Diego, USA.

10] Forslund C, Aspenberg P. Tendon healing stimulated by injected CDMP-2. Med Sci Sports Exerc 2001;33:685-687.

11] Forslund C, Aspenberg P. Improved healing of transected rabbit Achilles tendon after a single injection of cartilage-derived morphogenetic protein-2. Am J Sports Med 2003;31:555-559.

12] Forslund C, Bylander B, Aspenberg P. Indomethacin and celecoxib improve tendon healing in rats. Acta Orthop Scand 2003a;74:465-469.

13] Forslund C, Rueger D and Aspenberg P. A comparative dose-response study of cartilage-derived morphogenetic protein (CDMP)-1, -2 and -3 for tendon healing in rats. J Orthop Res 2003b;21:617-621.

14] Forrester JC, Zederfeldt BH, Hayes TL, Hunt TK. Wolff's law in relation to the healing skin wound. Journal of Trauma-Injury Infection & Critical Care 1970;10:770-779.

15] Gelberman RH, Botte MJ, Spiegelman JJ, Akeson WH. The excursion and deformation of repaired flexor tendons treated with protected early motion. Journal of Hand Surgery - American Volume 1986;11:106-110.

16] Greenlee TK Jr., Pike D. Studies of tendon healing in the rat. Remodelling of the distal stump after severance. Plastic & Reconstructive Surgery 1971;48:260-270.

17] Lundborg G, Rank F. Experimental studies on cellular mechanisms involved in healing of animal and human flexor tendon in synovial environment. [In Vitro. Journal Article] Hand 1980;12:3-11.

18] Magra M, Maffulli N. Nonsteroidal antiinflammatory drugs in tendinopathy: friend or foe. Clin J Sport Med 2006;16:1-3.

19] Mammoto T, Seerattan RA, Paulson KD, Leonard CA, Bray RC, Salo PT. Nerve growth factor improves ligament healing. J Orthop Res 2008 Feb 26 [Epub ahead of print].

20] Martin P. Wound healing--aiming for perfect skin regeneration. Science 1997; 276:75-81.

21] Potenza A. Critical Evaluation of Flexor-Tendon Healing and Adhesion Formation within Artificial Digital Sheaths: an experimental study.
J. Bone Joint Surg Am1963; 45: 1217-1233.

22] Rickert M, Jung M, Adiyaman M, Richter W, Simank H G. A growth and differentiation factor-5 (GDF-5)-coated suture stimulates tendon healing in an Achilles tendon model in rats. Growth Factors 2001;19:115-126.

23] Schepull T, Kvist A and Aspenberg P. Mechanical properties during healing of Achilles tendon ruptures predict final outcome. A Roentgen stereophotogrammetric analysis in 10 patients. BMC Musculoskeletal Disorders 2007;8:1-16.

24] Steyaert AE, Burssens PJ, Vercruysse CW, Vanderstraeten GG, Verbeeck RM. The effects of substance P on the biomechanic properties of ruptured rat Achilles' tendon. Arch Phys Med Rehabil 2006;87:254-258.

25] Strickland J. Flexor tendon injuries I: Foundations of treatment. Journal of the American Academy of Orthopaedic Surgeons 1995;3:55-62.

26] Takai S, Woo SL, Horibe S, Tung DK, Gelberman RH. The effects of frequency and duration of controlled passive mobilization on tendon healing. Journal of Orthopaedic Research 1991; 9:705-713.

27] Virchenko O, Aspenberg P. How can one platelet injection after tendon injury lead to a stronger tendon after 4 weeks? Interplay between early regeneration and mechanical stimulation. Acta Orthop 2006;77:806-812.

28] Virchenko O, Fahlgren A, Skoglund B, Aspenberg P. CDMP-2 injection improves early tendon healing in a rabbit model for surgical repair. Scand J Med Sci Sports 2005;15:260-264.

29] Virchenko O, Grenegard M, Aspenberg P. Independent and additive stimulation of tendon repair by thrombin and platelets. Acta Orthop 2006;77:960-966.

30] Virchenko O, Lindahl T, Aspenberg P. Low Molecular Weight Heparin impairs tendon repair. J Bone Joint Surg (B) 2007;in press.

31] Virchenko O, Skoglund B, Aspenberg P. Parecoxib impairs early tendon repair but improves later remodeling. Am J Sports Med 2004;32:1743-1747.

"Treat the patient, not the X-ray."

(James M. Hunter)

CHAPTER 4.

DIAGNOSIS

Aimee C. Stroink, H. Thermann

Take Home Message

• The Achilles tendon rupture is diagnosed clinically. It should be based on thorough clinical examination, including palpation, the calf squeeze test and a single leg heel rise.
• In doubtful or partial rupture cases, dynamic ultrasonography can be performed to confirm the diagnosis.

Introduction

Overuse and traumatic injuries of the Achilles tendon are among the most common tendinous abnormalities in the body, accounting for 20% of all running injuries and 9% of all ballet injuries[5]. The diagnosis 'acute Achilles tendon rupture' is made by means of clinical examination.

Additional investigation, such as plain radiographs, ultrasonography, and Magnetic Resonance Imaging (MRI) can be performed to exclude any bony pathology or to confirm the diagnosis in doubtful cases.

Physical examination

Normally, patients report sudden intense pain in the distal portion of the Achilles tendon, and often state that something or somebody might have struck their heel. On clinical examination, a positive calf squeeze test and a gap in the Achilles tendon, most often 3 to 6 cm above the insertion on the calcaneus, is consistently found. The most striking sign is the inability to perform a single heel rise in patients with acute as well as chronic Achilles tendon ruptures.

In 1976, Nillius and co-workers investigated the incidence of the Achilles tendon rupture; they found that 25% of the Achilles tendon ruptures were initially missed by the first evaluating physician[16]. Although this study is often cited, it is hardly representative, neither in terms of the difficulties of diagnosing the rupture nor concerning the diagnostic skills of the (orthopaedic) surgeons and residents. The false negative diagnosis can be due to difficulties in the differential diagnosis of a total or partial rupture, a "tennis-leg", a traumatic haematoma of the lower leg, an avulsion fracture of the calcaneus, a bursitis, or Achilles tendinopathy[2].
Physical examination can be equivocal, given the presence of some active plantarflexion, from the action to the posterior tibial tendon, the peroneal tendons and the long toe flexors. However, this will never be sufficient for single leg heel-raise.
The various physical tests (and their statistic values) are listed in table 1[14].
Another potential for diagnostic difficulties is due to delay of presentation, the interval between injury and examination, the swelling due to oedema and haematoma, which may obscure the findings on palpation[2,4,7].

Palpation	A gap in the Achilles tendon, most often 3 to 6 cm above the insertion in the calcaneus. (sensitivity 0.73, specificity 0.89)
Single leg heel rise	The patient is asked to perform a single leg heel rise. If the patient is able to lift his or her heel against gravity, the Achilles tendon is not ruptured.
Calf squeeze test	Also known as the Simmond's or Thompson's test. The patient lies prone with both feet hanging from the examination table. The examiner squeezes the affected calf muscle; if the Achilles tendon is intact, the foot will plantarflex. If the Achilles tendon is ruptured, the foot will remain in the resting position, or only minimal plantarflexion will occur. On the affected side, the calf muscle should be squeezed at the level where the largest range of motion will be reached on the healthy side. (sensitivity 0.96, specificity 0.93)

Knee flexion test	This was described by Matles. The patient lies prone, and is asked to flex both knees to 90°. During this movement, the position of both ankles is observed. An Achilles tendon rupture is diagnosed if the foot of the affected limb falls into neutral or dorsiflexion. If the tendon is intact, the foot will remain slightly plantarflexed. (sensitivity 0.88, specificity 0.85)
Sphygmomanometer test	Also known as Copeland's test. The patient lies prone with both feet extending the examination table. The ankle is passively plantarflexed, a sphygmomanometer cuff is placed halfway up the calf, and inflated to 100 mmHg. Subsequently, the examiner dorsiflexes the ankle. No pressure rise will be seen if the tendon is ruptured. If the Achilles tendon is intact, however, a pressure rise of 35-60 mmHg is measured. (sensitivity 0.78)
Needle test	Also known as O'Brien's test. The patient lies prone with both feet hanging from the examination table. Just medial to the midline, 10 cm proximal to the superior border of the calcaneus,

Table 1: Physical examination tests[14]

Imaging

If any diagnostic doubt still exists after a clear history and physical examination, the next step is to perform ultrasonography (US) of the Achilles tendon and its insertion.
High-frequency probes improve the imaging capacity of the degenerative changes, but for a rupture a 5-7.5 MHz probe is sufficient.
At US, the tendon should be examined in both longitudinal and axial planes[3]. An acute tendon rupture mostly appears as a focal lucency in the tendon, with a small amount of fluid in and surrounding the tendon. The frayed ends of the tendons can be detected, and they separate in dorsiflexion. In 75% of acute cases, a nearly complete juxtaposition of the stumps can be seen. In dorsiflexion, a visible gap can be shown in patients with a complete rupture. In partial ruptures, the proximal gliding of the tendon and tendon muscle unit can be depicted. In plantarflexion, full juxtaposition of the tendon stumps has been used as a basis for non-operative treatment can be assessed[18,19]. In delayed ruptures, complete juxtaposition is not possible, and an echogenic clot (haematoma) is seen between the tendon stumps, even in plantar flexion.

Ultrasonography is effective in differentiating synovial thickening from fluid around the tendon. As a rule of thumb, in a healthy tendon, the amount of fluid in the tendon sheath or a thickening is not visible.

US can be of additional value in localising the tendon ends when surgery is planned. This might assist the surgical procedure when small incisions are used in case of a large haematoma. The precise location of the tendon ends at a given position of flexion of the ankle should be noted in relation to the postero-superior corner of the calcaneus[3].

The other additional investigation is Magnetic Resonance Imaging (MRI). The sagittal images are most useful for differentiating pathologies of the Achilles tendon. The setting depends on the differential diagnosis. The T1-weighted images will provide anatomic details, whereas T2-weighted images are useful to evaluate the alterations in water content[5].
The average thickness of the Achilles tendon is approximately 6 mm, and 1 mm slices in the sagittal plane are mandatory to accurately depict the pathology.
The normal retrocalcaneal area is visible at MR imaging, and should be at most 6 mm (superior to inferior), 3 mm (medial to lateral), and 2 mm (anterior to posterior).
In comparison with ultrasonography, conventional MRI is less valuable in differentiating synovial thickening from free fluid. A superior image will be obtained by injecting Gadolinium DTPA, which increases the signal within most areas of synovitis. Internal splits and tears can be clearly seen as lines on T1-weighted images and/or oedema within the tendon on T2[3].
In complete Achilles tendon rupture with retraction, MRI will demonstrate a tendon gap with fraying of the tendon ends[12]. In acute ruptures, the tendon gap demonstrates intermediate signal on T1- and hyperintensity, oedema and haemorrhage, on T2-weighted images. In chronic ruptures, the tendon may be replaced by scar or fat tissue[15].

A diagnostic pitfall can be a heterogeneous area from the presence of connective tissue with intratendinous vessels between the collagen bundles. On T1-weighted and gradient echo images, it results in punctuate and short linear hyperintense foci[8]. This heterogeneity is given by the confluence of the gastrocnemius and soleus tendon into the Achilles tendon, and is normal. It can be distinguished from partial rupture, because the tendon demonstrates no morphological changes, and maintains its flat-to-concave anterior surface on axial MR images.

Plain radiological examinations have their main value in diagnosing an avulsion rupture, Haglund's deformity, or any other bony pathology at the tuber calcaneii.

The most important difference between ultrasonography and MRI is the possibility of dynamic examination in dorsiflexion and plantarflexion[18,19]. Partial tendon tears will not separate on ankle movement, and the tendon ends will not show paradoxical movement[3].

Conclusion

The patient's history and a thorough clinical examination, with at least palpation, the calf squeeze test and a single heel rise, are the most decisive tools to establish an Achilles tendon rupture.

The advantages of ultrasonography, such as dynamic assessment potential, wide availability, favourable time and cost factors, are important considerations to select an ultrasound examination as the first additional step to establish an acute Achilles tendon rupture in doubtful cases. MRI shows greater detail on the extent of tendon degeneration[17], but is hardly ever indicated in the diagnostic evaluation of acute Achilles tendon ruptures.

Imaging examinations should not be used routinely to diagnose acute Achilles tendon ruptures, and are probably overused, with the consequence that multiple normal anatomic variants may be erroneously interpreted as pathological. Familiarity of the examiner with normal anatomic variants is important for accurate diagnostic interpretation of ultrasonography and MR images.

References

1] Alfredson H, Pietilä T, Öhberg L, Lorentzon R. Achilles tendinosis and calf muscle strength.The effect of short-term immobilization after surgical treatment. Am J Sports Med 1998;26:166-171.

2] Arner O, Lindholm A. Subcutaneous rupture of the Achilles tendon; a study of 92 cases. Acta Chir Scand 1959;Suppl 11:1-51.

3] Baert AL, Knauth M, Sartor K. Injuries of the Ligament and Tendons in the Ankle and Foot. Imaging of orthopedic sports injuries. Ed. Vanhoenacker FM, Maas M, Gielen JL. Springer, 2007.

4] Beltran J et al. Tendons: high-field-strength, surface coil MR imaging. Radiol 1987:162;735-740.

5] Bencardino JT, Rosenberg ZS, Serrano LF. MR imaging of tendon abnormalities of the foot and ankle. Magn Reson Imaging Clin N Am 2001;9: 475-492.

6] Bleakney RR, White LM. Imaging of the Achilles tendon. Foot Ankle Clin 2005;10:239-254.

7] Daffner RH et al. Magnetic resonance imaging in acute tendon ruptures. Skeletal Radiol 1986;15:619-621.

8] Dussault RG, Kaplan PA, Roederer G. MR imaging of Achilles tendon in patients with familial hyperlipidemia: Comparison with plain films, physical examination, and patients with traumatic tendon lesions. AJR Am J Roentgenol 1995;164:403-407. Discussion of findings obtained by computed tomography and morphologic studies. Am J Sports Med 1979;7:121-126.

9] Grechenig W et al. The value of ultrasonography of the Achilles tendon in traumatology. Radiologe 1997;37:322-329.

10] Jahs MH. Tendon Disorders of the Foot and Ankle. Philadelphia: WB Saunders, 1991.

11] Kayser R, Mahlfeld K, Heyde CE. Partial rupture of the proximal Achilles tendon: a differential diagnostic problem in ultrasound imaging. Br J Sports Med 2005;39:838-842.

12] Keene JS et al. Magnetic-Resonance Imaging of Achilles-Tendon Ruptures. Am J Sports Med 1989;17:333-337.

13] Knobloch K, Thermann H, Huefner T. Dynamic ultrasound as a selection tool for reducing Achilles tendon ruptures. Am J Sports Med 2007;35:150.

14] Maffulli N. The clinical diagnosis of subcutaneous tear of the Achilles Tendon. Am J Sports Med 1998;26:266-270.

15] Marcus DS, Reicher MA, Kellerhouse LE. Achilles-Tendon Injuries - the Role of Mr Imaging. J Comp Ass Tomography 1989;13:480-486.

16] Nillius SA, Nilsson BE, Westlin NE. The incidence of Achilles tendon rupture. Acta Orthop Scand 1976;47:118-121.

17] Robson MD et al. Magnetic resonance imaging of the Achilles tendon using ultrashort TE (UTE) pulse sequences. Clin Radiol 2004;59: 727-735.

18] Thermann H, Foffmann R, Zwipp H, Tscherne H. The use of ultrasonography in the foot and ankle. Foot and Ankle 1992;13: 386-390.

19] Thermann H, Zwipp H, Tscherne H. Functional treatment concept of acute rupture of the Achilles tendon. 2 years results of a prospective randomized study. Unfallchirurg 1995;98:21-32.

"Faith and knowledge lean largely upon each other in the practice of medicine."

(Peter Mere Latham)

CHAPTER 5.

OVERVIEW OF REVIEWS

Maayke N. van Sterkenburg, C. Niek van Dijk

Take Home Message

• *Management of acute Achilles tendon rupture should be adjusted to the patient's lifestyle. Conservative management leads to higher rerupture rates, and surgical treatment to higher complication rates other than rerupture.*
• *Postoperative functional bracing leads to a shorter rehabilitation period when compared to immobilisation in a cast.*
• *Subjective outcome scores are recommended to be used as a primary outcome measure.*

1. Introduction

'Rupture of the Achilles tendon should be operated on without delay' (Quénu and Stoianovitch, 1929)
'Operative repair of Achilles tendon rupture is unnecessary' (Lea and Smith, 1972)

There is a lack of consensus concerning the best management of the acute Achilles tendon rupture. Operative management is typically reserved for high-demand patients, while the sedentary are treated conservatively in cast.

2. Overview of systematic reviews

2.1. Lo and co-workers (1997)[10]

Lo and co-workers performed a quantitative review on surgical versus non-surgical treatment. They identified 2 prospective randomized trials and 17 case series and concluded that no clear recommendations could be made. The rerupture rate for surgical operative management was found to be substantially lower compared with non-surgical management at the expense of the minor and moderate complication rate of operative management, which was 20 times greater. They concluded that patients with poor healing potential should be treated non-surgically, and active patients should be offered both surgical and non-surgical management.

2.2. Wong and co-workers (2002)[25]

Wong and co-workers identified 125 studies. 83 Of these studies were retrospective, there were 20 prospective studies, 18 retrospective comparative studies, and only 4 were randomized controlled trials. All compared surgical intervention in cast or functional after-treatment with non-surgical management in cast or functional brace. The complications described in each study were divided into three categories: wound complications (major/minor), general complications (major/minor) and rerupture.

The patients managed non-surgically generally underwent a period of immobilisation in a below-the-knee cast in the gravity equines position for 4 weeks, and with the ankle placed in a more neutral position for an additional 4 weeks. Three studies described management purely by functional bracing. All reported good functional outcome and low rerupture rates. The average time of immobilisation in these studies was only 2 weeks. Of the 645 patients who underwent non-surgical management, there were 55 (8.5%) who sustained minor general complications, 4 (0.6%) with major complications, and 63 (9.8%) who experienced rerupture.

Two-hundred and forty-seven patients underwent percutaneous repair (different techniques) and immobilisation, and 122 patients underwent percutaneous repair and early mobilisation. In percutaneous techniques, entrapment of the sural nerve is relatively common.
Of the 247 patients in the immobilized group, the number of minor wound complications reported was 12 (4.9%), the general complication rate was 21 (8.5%) minor and 2 (0.8%) major complications, and there were 9 (3.6%) reruptures. The 122 patients in the early-mobilized group sustained 8 (6.6%) minor and 4 (3.3%) major wound complications, 18 (14.8%) minor and 1 (0.8%) major general complication, and there were 8 (6.6%) reruptures.

Many different open methods of repair have been described. There were 3718 Achilles tendon ruptures managed with open repair and immobilization, and 283

Achilles tendon ruptured managed with open repair and early mobilization (table 1). Of the 3718 patients managed with open repair and immobilization, there were 457 (12.3%) minor and 86 (2.3%) major wound complications, 301 (8.1%) minor and 29 (0.8%) major general complications and 82 (2.2%) reruptures. Of the 283 patients managed with open repair and early mobilization, there were 14 (4.9%) minor and 1 (0.4%) major wound complication, 15 (5.3%) minor and 1 (0.4%) major general complication, and 4 (1.4%) reruptures.

Complications/ Achilles tendon rupture management	Conservative management	Percutaneous repair: Immobilisation	Percutaneous repair[1]: Early mobilisation	Open surgery[2]: Immobilisation	Open surgery[2]: Early mobilisation
N	645	247	122	3718	283
Minor wound	-	12 (4.9%)	8 (6.6%)	457 (12.3%)	14 (4.9%)
Major wound	-	-	4 (3.3%)	86 (2.3%)	1 (0.4%)
Minor general	55 (8.5%)	21 (8.5%)	18 (14.8%)	301 (8.1%)	15 (4.9%)
Major general	4 (0.6%)	2 (0.8%)	1 (0.8%)	29 (0.8%)	1 (0.4%)
Rerupture	63 (9.8%)	9 (3.6%)	8 (6.6%)	82 (2.2%)	4 (1.4%)

Table 1: Complications

[2]At least 4 different percutaneous techniques were used
[2]The preferred method for early-diagnosed ruptures has been simple end-to-end suture, but collected data revealed that 41 different open techniques were used.

Wong and co-workers found that, in general, the number of publications reporting Achilles tendon ruptures was increasing, and the trend for the number of reported complications was decreasing. Few studies used standardised subjective scoring to assess patient satisfaction and recovery after an Achilles tendon rupture.
In conclusion, the published studies showed a trend toward earlier mobilization. Open repair followed by early mobilisation gives the best functional recovery at an acceptable complication rate.

2.3. Bhandari and co-workers (2002)[2]

Bhandari and co-workers published the results of a quantitative systematic review of only randomized and quasi-randomized trials to determine the effect of surgical versus conservative management of acute Achilles tendon ruptures on the rate of rerupture. Computerized databases were searched to locate published clinical studies and results of this meta-analysis were compared with recommendations in the literature.
Pooled analysis of 5 studies with 421 patients revealed a non-significant difference in the proportion of patients who regained normal function after surgical

or non-surgical management (71% versus 63%, respectively). Similarly, analysis of six studies with 448 patients did not reveal any difference in the risk of sponta-neous complaints (heel aches with walking, increased shoe size because of wid-ening of the Achilles tendon and ankle stiffness) at follow-up between surgical repair and non-surgically treated groups (19% versus 25% respectively).

Apart from this pooled analysis, Bhandari and co-workers studied recommenda-tions with regards to the management of Achilles tendon ruptures which were made in 22 review articles and textbooks. They found that 16 authors strongly favoured surgery (72.7%); four were noncommittal (18.2%), and two strongly fa-voured conservative therapy (9.1%).

According to Bhandari and co-workers, the most obvious drawback to surgical intervention is the increased risk of infection. In the current group of trials, there was a 4.7% incidence of infection after surgery and no infections after conserva-tive management. Wound slough may occur at a rate of 0.85%, and sural nerve injury at a rate of 6% after operative repair. Deep venous thrombosis is more common after non-surgical management of Achilles tendon ruptures (1.5%).

Bhandari and co-workers postulated that strong recommendations require a large, randomized trial comparing surgery and conservative therapy for acute Achilles tendon ruptures.

2.4 Kocher and co-workers (2002)[9]

Kocher and co-workers performed an expected-value decision analysis to de-termine the optimal management strategy for management of acute Achilles tendon rupture, whether surgical or non-surgical. Included were randomized controlled trials, cohort studies and case series; 25 studies reporting data on operative management and 10 studies reporting data concerning non-surgical management were evaluated.

COMPLICATIONS	Major	Moderate	Minor
	Re-rupture	sural nerve injury	adhesion of the
	Second re-rupture	wound problems	scar
	Tendon lengthening	not requiring	
	Deep infection	reoperation	
	Chronic fistula		
	DVT		
	(pulmonary embolus)		

Table 2: Complications described

As in the review by Wong and co-workers, the severity of complications was di-vided into 3 groups (Table 2).

This systematic review revealed that the probability of rerupture after non-surgical management was 12.1%, whereas the rerupture rate after surgical repair was only 2.2%. However, the probability of a moderate (mainly wound) complication after surgical repair was 7.5% versus 0.3% from conservative management. As in the three former reviews, this investigation also found that surgical management was the optimal management strategy for acute Achilles tendon rupture. Results in terms of return to work time and rate to return to the previous level of sports participation were summarized, but no conclusions were drawn.

Like Bhandari and co-workers, Kocher and co-workers also described the fact that variations in specific management regimens existed within the two treatment arms2. Furthermore, they did not study percutaneous repair since there were insufficient data.

In conclusion, Kocher and co-workers advocated a model of shared decision-making in which the physician and the patient are jointly involved in the medical decision-making process.

2.5 Lynch and co-workers (2003)[12]

Lynch and co-workers performed a comprehensive literature search to retrieve relevant English language articles comparing surgical with non-surgical management. They identified 5 prospective randomized controlled trials between 1966 and 2002.

The outcomes assessed were not only re-rupture rate and complications, but also plantar flexion strength, interval to return to work, and level of sporting activity attained post-treatment. A definition of the goals of management in spontaneous Achilles tendon ruptures put forward by McComis and co-workers was used, namely to restore tendon length and tension, to optimise ultimate strength and function, to reduce the time needed for rehabilitation and to facilitate an early return to work and to pre-injury level of activity[14].

Lynch and co-workers also found that there is a lack of a universal, consistent protocol for subjective and objective evaluation following treatment, which renders the comparison of results difficult. In their opinion, from the available evidence, surgical management is preferable to non-surgical management because it produces better functional outcome.

As did the former 4 reviewers, Lynch and co-workers found that the incidence of rerupture following non-surgical management is significantly higher than after surgical management; only 5 patients need to be treated surgically to prevent one re-rupture. This higher rate may be associated with ankle positioning in inadequate plantar flexion during immobilisation.

The incidence of minor complications following surgical management is substantial, but these do not appear to affect functional outcome. Return to sport at one year, reduction in active plantar flexion, increased dorsiflexion, isokinetic strength or endurance testing revealed no significant differences.

Postoperative early functional mobilisation is more acceptable to patients than plaster cast immobilisation, and also results in improved functional outcomes such as increased ROM and earlier return to pre-injury level of activity, probably because early motion helps to align the collagen fibres, thereby improving tensile strength and gliding ability.

Lynch and co-workers conclude that non-surgical management should be reserved for patients who refuse or who are unfit for operative repair. In the end, patients should be consulted regarding their management preference.

2.6. Khan and co-workers (2005)[7]

Khan and co-workers performed a meta-analysis trying to identify and summarise the evidence from randomised controlled trials on the effectiveness of different interventions in the management of acute Achilles tendon ruptures. The authors searched multiple databases and the reference lists of articles, and contacted the authors of the various studies. Twelve trials involving 800 patients were included. The primary outcomes were complications of management and rerupture. Other outcomes, such as the level of sporting activity, patient satisfaction, and the length of hospital stay, were omitted because they lacked quantity and uniformity to support rigorous meta-analysis. Five comparisons were made.

2.6.1. Open surgical versus non-surgical management

This comparison concerns 4 trials comparing open surgical to non-surgical management, which included a total of 356 patients. There was a lower risk of rerupture in surgically managed patients (3.5 % versus 12.6% in nonoperatively treated patients), with a higher risk of other complications including infection, adhesions and disturbed skin sensibility (34.1% versus 2.7%).

2.6.2. Post-operative splinting: cast immobilisation versus cast immobilisation followed by functional bracing

This was considered in 5 studies. Rerupture rates were reported in five studies, but none found a statistically significant difference. Also five studies commented upon complications of management. The pooled rate of rerupture was 5.0% (7/150) in the cast immobilization group and 2.3% (3/133) in the functional brace group. The pooled incidence of reported complications other than rerupture was 50/140 (35.7%) in the cast immobilised group and 26/133 (19.5%) in the functional brace group.

2.6.3. Open surgical versus percutaneous repair

Two studies included 94 patients. The rerupture rate in open surgery was 4.3% and 2.1% using a percutaneous technique. Complication rates other than rerupture in open surgery were 26.1% and 8.3% in percutaneous repair. The pooled rate of reported complications (excluding rerupture) was 26.1% in the open group and 8.3% in the percutaneous group. The pooled rate of infection was 19.6% in the open group and 0% in the percutaneous group.

2.6.4. Postoperative splinting: in cast alone versus splinting in a cast followed by functional bracing

Data from 273 patients were available in 5 studies. The rerupture rate in cast immobilisation was 5.0% versus 2.3% in functional bracing. Other complications with cast immobilisation rated 35.7% versus 19.5% with functional bracing (adhesions, altered sensibility, keloid or scar hypertrophy).

2.6.5. Comparing different non-surgical management regimens (cast versus functional bracing)

Only 2 studies were identified, including 90 patients. Because of the small number of patients involved no definitive conclusions could be drawn with regards to different non-surgical management regimes. The authors also reported a difference in regimen and minimal reporting of outcomes. The rerupture rate treating patients with a functional brace was 2.4%, compared with 12.2% in the casting group.

This meta-analysis concluded that non-surgically managed patients have more than 3 times higher risk of rerupture but have a minimal risk of other complications whereas one-third of surgically treated patients have a complication.
There is a tendency towards a lower grade of complications, including infections, in the percutaneously treated patients.
Postoperative management favours the outcome of functional bracing instead of cast alone. Different regimens of postoperative splinting in a cast followed by a functional brace reduce the overall complication rate.

3. Discussion

Between 1981 and 2005, 14 different randomized controlled trials were published on the management of acute Achilles tendon ruptures. These trials have been the focus of 6 systematic reviews that were published between 1997 and 2005 (table 3). Of the 14 trials, 4 were quasi-randomized[6,10,13,21] and in 5 studies the method of randomization was not described [3,4,17,24,25]. Because of these flaws these systematic reviews have not been consistent in their analysis. Bhandari[2] was very strict in his inclusion criteria and included only 3 randomized trials while Khan included 12[7]. (table 3)

REVIEW / RCT	Lo (1997)	Wong (2002)	Bhandari (2002)	Kocher (2002)	Lynch (2003)	Khan (2005)
Nistor (1981)	√	√	√	√	√	√
Mortensen (1992)	√[1]	√	X[2]	√[1]	X[2]	X[2]
Saleh (1992)	?	√	X[7]	?	√	√
Cetti (1993)	√	√	√	√[1]	√	√
Cetti (1994)	√[1]	?	X[3,5]	√	?	√
Mortensen (1996)	?[4/6]	?[4]	?[4]	?[4]	?[4]	X[6]
Schroeder (1997)		?[4/5]	?[4/5]	?[4/5]	?[4/5]	√
Mortensen (1999)		?	X[8]	√[1]	√	√
Möller (2001)			√	√	√	√
Lim (2001)						√
Petersen (2002)						√
Kerkhoffs (2002)						√
Maffulli (2003)						√
Kangas (2003)						√
TOTAL 14						

Table 3: This table shows all randomized controlled trials (RCT) that were analyzed in the six systematic reviews

√ = RCT used in analysis
X = not used, reason described
? = RCT not used for unknown reason.

[1] Included in this review as a case series, not as a randomized prospective trial.

[2] Excluded because the trial did not meet the inclusion criteria (it studies separation of tendon ends after Achilles tendon repair.)

[3] Excluded because of duplicate publication of data (Cetti 1993).

[4] Excluded because only the abstract of the trial was available and not the data.

[5] Excluded because this study did not adequately describe randomisation.

[6] Excluded because this study is unique, comparing below-the-knee with above-the-knee cast after Achilles tendon repair.

[7] Excluded because the trial did not meet the inclusion criteria (it compares the Sheffield splint for controlled early mobilisation after rupture of the calcaneal tendon to cast immobilisation)

[8] Excluded because the trial did not meet the inclusion criteria (it investigates early motion of the ankle after Achilles tendon repair)

Apart from the above-mentioned 14 randomized controlled trials, several cohort studies and case series have been published. Four reviewers mixed the outcome of randomized controlled trials with case series and cohort studies (see APPENDIX for an extensive description of in- and exclusion criteria developed by all six reviewers), which makes them more open to bias. Lo included 15 case series and 4 randomized trials[11]. Wong included 125 studies, of which 83 were retrospective, 20 were prospective and 18 were retrospective comparative studies[27]. Only 4 were randomized controlled trials (table 3). Bhandari only included randomized and quasi-randomized trials (table 3)[2]. Kocher[9] included 35 studies according to the inclusion criteria described by Lo and co-workers[11]. Lynch also included nonrandomized trials; 16 studies were included of which 5 were randomized trials (table 3), 6 comparative studies and 5 were reviews 12. Khan included quasi- randomized and randomized studies, but also studies that stated they were randomized but did not describe the method of randomization (table 3)[7].

The outcomes of the reviews that included nonrandomized studies are open to bias. Some of these generated more detailed results because data on larger amounts of patients and more diverse outcome measures were available for analysis. Wong, for example, included 125 studies and therefore was able to describe complications in much more detail than Bhandari, who found it hard to make a solid recommendation from the small amount of studies available[2,27]. Despite the inclusion of non-randomized trials and therefore a larger amount of studies in some reviews, we did not find any significant contradictions in the outcome of reviews which included data from non-randomized trials and reviews that did not. Because of probable bias, results from reviews including nonrandomized studies are hard to interpret and valid conclusions cannot be drawn. We investigated the reviews on argumentation to include one randomized trial and exclude the other. Khan and co-workers[7] included 12 of 14 retrieved trials, regardless of unclear or un-stated randomization. They also included a trial performed by Schroeder[25], although only the abstract was available. Lo and co-workers included 2 randomized controlled trials and 17 case series[11]. They classified 2 trials as being case series[4,16], while these trials should have been classified as being randomized trials (table 3). This means that they included 4 randomized trials. The trial performed by Saleh and co-workers[24] is probably excluded because randomisation was not stated. Wong and co-workers[27] included 4 studies, but they did not retrieve 2 other randomized trials available (Mortensen and co-workers, Saleh and co-workers)[16,24], possibly because in the trial by Saleh and co-workers randomisation was not stated, and because the study by Mortensen and co-workers was available only as an abstract (table 3).

From the 9 trials available, Bhandari and co-workers[2] included 3 of 4 studies comparing surgical with non-surgical management[3,15,21]. Schroeder was not included, because only the abstract was available. Bhandari and co-workers[2] stated that Cetti 1994 was a duplicate publication of data from Cetti 1993, and therefore excluded Cetti 1994[3,4]. We have not been able to confirm this. Cetti 1993 compares surgical with non-surgical management in a group of patients included from October 1982 to May 1984[3], whereas Cetti 1994 compares postoperative management in a rigid cast with postoperative management in a mobile cast in a group of patients included from September 1985 to November 1986[4]. Both groups are clearly different, and it is unlikely that data were duplicated.

Kocher[9] performed article inclusion according to the criteria of Lo and co-workers[11] and retrieved 3 randomized controlled trials. As in the study of Lo and co-workers, Kocher and co-workers also included case series in their review, and labelled 3 randomized trials as being case series[9]. Both reviews included Cetti 1993 and 1994, where and co-workers included Cetti 1993 as being a randomized trial, and Cetti 1994 as a case series; Kocher and co-workers included Cetti 1993 as a case series and Cetti 1994 as a randomized trial[3,4]. Also, a case series published by Nistor in 1976 on non-surgical management of acute Achilles tendon ruptures was erroneously included as a randomized trial[20]. Because both case series and cohort studies were also included in the analysis performed by Kocher and co-workers[9], this probably did not have further implications. The study of Saleh and co-workers[24] was not included for unknown reasons.

Lynch and co-workers[12] only included randomized trials comparing surgical with non-surgical management, functional immobilisation and immobilisation in a cast in both surgical and non-surgical management. Cetti 1994 and Schroeder 1997 were not mentioned in his study, probably because they were not retrieved, or they did not meet the criteria of comparative studies mentioned above[4,25].

In conclusion, some reviewers erroneously included non-randomized trials, and some excluded trials that were adequately randomized. Despite these flaws, we did not find any significant contradictions in the outcome of the reviews performed.

Few randomised controlled studies reported outcome measures such as length of hospital stay, time to return to work, time to return to sport, level of sports activity post- rupture, calf circumference or muscle atrophy, tendon elongation, power/strength- testing, range of motion, pain and patient satisfaction. Two out of six reviewers tried to pool these outcomes, but found inconsistent and insufficient results (table 4). From the patient's point of view, these outcome measures are probably more important than rerupture rate, wound complications and infection, which can be unpleasant complications, but, in most instances, can be successfully managed.

AUTHOR	RERUPTURE RATE	WOUND COMPLICATIONS	GENERAL COMPLICATIONS	OTHER (return to work/sports/ satisfaction etc.)
Lo (1997)	√	√	√	-
Wong (2002)	√	√	√	-
Bhandari (2002)	√	√	-	√[1]
Kocher (2002)	√	√	√	-
Lynch (2003)	√	√	√	√[2]
Khan (2005)	√	√	√	-

Table 4: Outcome measures used for analysis

[1] All randomized and quasi-randomized trials that reported rerupture of the Achilles tendon were included. Secondary outcomes were defined as wound infections, return to normal function and (minor) complaints such as heel aches with walking, increased shoe size because of widening of the Achilles tendon and ankle stiffness. All relevant information from included studies was abstracted and pooled.

[2] Outcomes assessed were rerupture rate, major and minor complications, plantar flexion strength, interval to return to work, and level of sporting activity attained post-treatment. When sufficient data were available, relative risk reduction, absolute risk reduction, number needed to treat surgically to prevent one rerupture, and 95% confidence intervals were calculated.

Khan and co-workers performed a Cochrane Review in 2007, in which they included all 14 trials available, involving 891 patients[8]. This meta-analysis is similarly designed as his study from 2005[7], but now they also tried to pool data available on these mostly subjective outcomes. They found that no statistically significant differences were reported in the duration of in-hospital stay, but there was an expected trend for longer hospital-stay associated with surgery. Inconsistent results were reported for the duration of time off-work and level of sporting activities post-rupture and therefore no definite conclusions could be drawn for these outcome measures. Type of work performed (manual versus office-based) plays an important role in determining ones ability to return to employment, but this was only recorded in one study[15]. The methods used for reporting patient satisfaction was non-uniform and conflicting results were found between the studies. The best assessment was made by Möller, using Visual Analogue Scales (VAS)[13]. They reported that surgically managed patients had significantly better quality of life at 8 weeks and at 2 years post-rupture.

Two studies reported no difference in power of plantar flexion at follow-up. For other objective outcome measures such as range of motion and calf muscle atrophy, conflicting results were reported.

We feel that subjective outcome scores, as used by Möller are of great use to assess patients' outcome and to make recommendations based on the patients needs and complaints after Achilles tendon rupture.

4. Conclusion

In conclusion, no definitive recommendations can be made based on the literature published over the past 40 years. All reviewers suggest that management should be adjusted to the patients needs, that non-surgical management leads to higher rerupture rates and surgical management to higher complication rates other than rerupture. Most modern authors prefer post-operative functional bracing instead of long-term immobilisation in a cast.

Criteria for inclusion or exclusion of randomized controlled trials in the reviews we compared are clearly stated but often publications that could have been suitable for analysis were not retrieved or were excluded for unknown reason. Most reviewers included non-randomized studies which make the outcomes more prone to bias and therefore results are less reliable.

Concerning outcome, the focus thus far has been on rerupture rate and wound complications, which, although important, can usually be managed successfully. From the patient's point of view more important outcome parameters are pain, tendon elongation, range of motion, strength, hypotrophy and the possibility to return to sports. Secondary outcome measures such as work resumption, length of hospital stay, level of sport resumption and a temporary heel rise could be considered as well.

A subjective scoring system such as 'The Achilles Tendon Total Rupture Score' (ATRS), developed by Nilsson-Helander and co-workers[19], has been designed as a patient-reported instrument for measuring the outcome after surgical and non-surgical management of a complete Achilles tendon rupture. Also, the Foot and Ankle Outcome Score is a valid subjective scoring system. These questionnaires are recommended to be used in the assessment of patients with acute Achilles tendon rupture.

APPENDIX: Inclusion and exclusion criteria used in the six reviews

Lo and co-workers: A list of published studies was compiled, and the Medline Database and Index Medicus were searched. All retrieved articles were reviewed independently by at least three of four authors to decide on eligibility based on pre-determined criteria.

Exclusion criteria were: (1) injury is not a primary, acute spontaneous rupture of the Achilles tendon with no delay in treatment (defined as >4 weeks from rupture); (2) not a randomized clinical trial or cohort study with matching for major variables or case series in which it was expressly stated that there was no patient selection prior to treatment; (3) inability to extract data because treatment was not described in adequate detail; (4) review article; (5) data included in another published report; (6) treatment was considered experimental; (7) inability to extract data because the study was published in summary version only; (8) the report focused exclusively on patients who had special conditions, such as renal transplant.

Wong and co-workers: Each article was graded using a validated methods score developed by Tallon and co-workers[26]. Articles were also considered when published in French, German, Italian, or Spanish. All articles identified included the outcomes of studies reporting Achilles tendon ruptures. Also literature where randomization methods were not specified and non-randomized prospective studies were included.

Bhandari and co-workers: Articles that met the following criteria were included: (1) target population, individuals with an acute closed spontaneous rupture of the Achilles tendon; (2) intervention, surgical repair versus nonoperative treatment; (3) outcome, studies that reported rerupture of the Achilles tendon; and (4) methodological criterion, prospective, randomized trials.

Kocher and co-workers: Article inclusion was performed according to the criteria of Lo and co-workers.

Lynch and co-workers: Literature search was limited to adult patients and studies comparing surgical with non-surgical treatment of closed spontaneous ATR. Case reports were excluded. Validity of trials was assessed according to standard evidence-based guidelines for therapeutic trials, developed by Sackett and co-workers[23].

Khan and co-workers: All randomized and quasi-randomized trials comparing operative and nonoperative methods for the treatment of acute Achilles tendon ruptures were considered for inclusion. Trials were independently assessed for inclusion by four reviewers. Ten aspects of methodology were used to give a maximum score for each study of 12. In addition, risks of pre-allocation disclosure of assignment were rated according to the Cochrane Reviewer's Handbook[1]. Retrospective studies, studies with insufficient reporting of primary outcomes, studies with inadequate methods of randomization, and unique randomized controlled trials (where pooling of data was not possible) were excluded.

Acknowledgement

The financial support of the Stichting amphoraest (Foundation) is acknowledged.

Reference List

1] Alderson P, Green S, Higgins JPT, editors. Cochrane Reviewers' Handbook 4.2.1. The Cochrane Library, Issue 1, 2004.
2] Bhandari M, Guyatt GH, Siddiqui F, Morrow F, Busse J, Leighton RK, et al. Treatment of acute Achilles tendon ruptures: a systematic overview and metaanalysis. Clin Orthop Relat Res 2002:190-200.
3] Cetti R, Christensen S, Ejsted R, Jensen NM, Jorgensen U. Operative versus nonoperative treatment of Achilles tendon rupture: a prospective randomized study and review of the literature. Am J Sports Med 1993; 21:791-799.
4] Cetti R, Henriksen LO, Jacobsen KS. A new treatment of ruptured Achilles tendons. A prospective randomized study. Clin Orthop Relat Res 1994:155-165.
5] Kangas J, Pajala A, Siira P, Hamalainen M, Leppilahti J. Early functional treatment versus early immobilization in tension of the musculotendinous unit after Achilles rupture repair: a prospective, randomized, clinical study. J Trauma 2003 ;54:1171-1180.
6] Kerkhoffs GM, Struijs PA, Raaymakers EL, Marti RK. Functional treatment after surgical repair of acute Achilles tendon rupture: wrap vs walking cast. Arch Orthop Trauma Surg 2002;122:102-105.
7] Khan RJ, Fick D, Keogh A, Crawford J, Brammar T, Parker M. Treatment of acute achilles tendon ruptures. A meta-analysis of randomized, controlled trials. J Bone Joint Surg Am 2005;87:2202-2210.
8] Khan RJK, Fick D, Brammar TJ, Crawford J, Parker MJ. Surgical interventions for treating acute achilles tendon ruptures (review). The Cochrane Library 2007.
9] Kocher MS, Bishop J, Marshall R, Briggs KK, Hawkins RJ. Operative versus nonoperative management of acute Achilles tendon rupture: expected-value decision analysis. Am J Sports Med 2002;30:783-790.
10] Lim J, Dalal R, Waseem M. Percutaneous versus open repair of the ruptured Achilles tendon: a prospective randomized controlled study. Foot Ankle Int 2001; 22:559-568.
11] Lo IK, Kirkley A, Nonweiler B, Kumbhare DA. Operative versus nonoperative treatment of acute Achilles tendon ruptures: a quantitative review. Clin J Sport Med 1997;7:207-211.
12] Lynch RM. Achilles tendon rupture: surgical versus non-surgical treatment. Accid Emerg Nurs 2004;12:149-158.
13] Maffulli N, Tallon C, Wong J, Lim KP, Bleakney R. Early weightbearing and ankle mobilization after open repair of acute midsubstance tears of the achilles tendon. Am J Sports Med 2003;31:692-700.
14] McComis, Nawoczenski DA, DeHaven KE. Functional bracing for rupture of the Achilles tendon. Clinical results and analysis of ground-reaction forces and temporal data. J Bone Joint Surg Am 1997;79:1799-808.
15] Moller M, Movin T, Granhed H, Lind K, Faxen E, Karlsson J. Acute rupture of tendon Achillis. A prospective randomised study of comparison between surgical and non-surgical treatment. J Bone Joint Surg Br 2001;83:843-848.
16] Mortensen NH, Saether J, Steinke MS, Staehr H, Mikkelsen SS. Separation of tendon ends after achilles tendon repair: A prospective, randomized, multicenter study. Orthop 1992;15:899-903.
17] Mortensen NH, Sorensen L, Pless S. Below- knee versus above-knee cast after Achilles tendon repair- a prospective controlled trial (abstract). Act Orthop Scan. Suppl 1996;67:38.
18] Mortensen HM, Skov O, Jensen PE. Early motion of the ankle after operative treatment of a rupture of the Achilles tendon. A prospective, randomized clinical and radiographic study. J Bone Joint

Surg Am 1999;81:983-990.

19] Nilsson-Helander K, Thomeé R, Grävare Silbernagel K, Thomeé P, Faxén E, Eriksson BI, Karlsson J. The Achilles tendon Total Rupture Score (ATRS): development and validation. Am J Sports Med 2007;35:421-426.

20] Nistor L. Conservative Treatment of Fresh Subcutaneous Rupture of the Achilles Tendon. Acta orthop scand 1976;47:459-462.

21] Nistor L. Surgical and non-surgical treatment of Achilles tendon rupture. J Bone Joint Surg 1981;63:394-399.

22] Petersen OF, Nielsen MB, Jensen KH, Solgaard S. CAM walker versus cast in conservative treatment of Achilles tendon rupture. Ugeskrift for Laeger 2002;164:3852-3855.

23] Sackett DL, Straus SE, Richardson WS, Rosenberg W, Haynes RB. Evidence-based Medicine, 2nd edition, Churchill Livingstone.

24] Saleh M, Marshall PD, Senoir R, MacFarlane A. The Sheffield splint for controlled early mobilisation after rupture of the calcaneal tendon. A prospective, randomized comparison with plaster treatment. J Bone Joint Surg Br 1992;74: 206-209.

25] Schroeder D, Lehmann M, Steinbrueck K. Treatment of acute achilles tendon ruptures: open vs. percutaneous repair vs. conservative treatment. A prospective randomized study (abstract). Orthop Trans 1997;21:1228.

26] Tallon C, Coleman B, Khan KM, Maffulli N. Outcome of surgery for chronic Achilles tendinopathy. Am J Sp Med 2001;29:315-320.

27] Wong J, Barrass V, Maffulli N. Quantitative review of operative and nonoperative management of Achilles tendon ruptures. Am J Sports Med 2002;30:565-575.

"The patient does not care about your
science; what he wants to know is,
can you cure him?"

(Martin H. Fischer)

Chapter 6.

OPEN SURGERY

Jon Karlsson, Maayke N. van Sterkenburg, Gino M.M.J. Kerkhoffs,
C. Niek van Dijk

Take Home Message

• *Open surgery is considered the standard procedure when operative manage-ment is contemplated in patients with acute Achilles tendon ruptures. All other operative management modalities (mini-invasive repair and percutaneous re-pair) should be compared with open surgery.*
• *The risk of rerupture after open end-to-end repair is low; however, there is a risk of other complications, such as adhesions and wound infections. This risk can be reduced by strict adherence to management protocols and patient compliance.*
• *Patients can start exercising ROM at 10 days post-operatively, or possibly earlier (immediately after the repair) as per patient's comfort. After 14 days weight-bear-ing with restricted dorsiflexion should be commenced.*

Introduction

The optimal management of Achilles tendon ruptures has long been debated. The discussions mainly focus on surgical versus non-surgical management. Even though the Achilles tendon is the strongest in the human body, it is one of the most commonly ruptured tendons. Most patients are middle-aged athletes. The rupture usually occurs 2 to 6 cm proximal to the insertion to the calcaneus, and the rupture ends are typically frayed. Whether the rupture happens in an area of tendinopathy or not is also a matter of debate. The injury most often happens suddenly, in patients who do not report tendon pain prior to the rupture. Most researchers suggest that typical tendinopathy does not precede an acute Achilles tendon rupture.

In most patients, patients report to have experienced a snapping sensation, and some thought that they had been kicked in the area of the Achilles tendon. A defect in the tendon is usually palpable and active plantarflexion is weakened. The calf squeeze test is positive. Imaging studies are not needed in most patients, although both MRI and high resolution real time ultrasonography can provide excellent information about the ruptured tendon. However, such studies are rarely needed to establish the diagnosis. Once the correct diagnosis has been clarified, appropriate management, either surgical or non-surgical, should be initiated. Controversy continues in terms of the optimal management, and not even randomized studies published during the last decade[9] are able to produce a clear and definitive management algorithm. Those authors who prefer surgical management do so as a rule due to less risk of rerupture after open surgery. Even though surgical management carries the risk of complications, such as wound breakdown, infection, thromboembolism, and stiffness, many patients are in favour of surgical management, given the lower risk of rerupture. A recent meta-analysis[5] reported a risk of rerupture of approximately 4-5% after surgical management and of approximately 13% after non-surgical management. This difference was counter-balanced by the increased risk of wound infections, up to 10% in some studies after surgical management. An important issue is the rehabilitation protocol after surgical management. An active rehabilitation program in a (removable) brace with early weight bearing has proven better than the immobilization in a cast[8,9]. For the conservatively treated patients, the issue of immobilization is also of concern. The trend is without doubt towards shorter immobilization and early range of motion training, e.g. (re)movable brace and early weight-bearing. In fact, it has been shown that early, well protected range of motion training and at least moderately aggressive rehabilitation will result in outcomes similar to surgical management[8].

Selection of surgical management modality

The important issue is when surgical management has been selected to make a choice of technique and approach. Repair can be performed using an open, minimally invasive or percutaneous approach. In this chapter, only the open approach will be discussed. We prefer to place the patient prone with their feet over a pillow or outside the operating table in order to avoid excessive plantar flexion, as over-tightening of the repair will result in (a higher risk of) tendon shortening and loss of motion. A soft roll can be placed under the tibia. The procedure can be carried out in general, regional, or local anaesthesia. A bloodless field is not needed. When considering the position of the foot, in order to avoid shortening or lengthening of the tendon, it is wise to compare the position to the other foot in neutral position. It is important to judge the tension of the repair and the balance between the dorsi- and the plantar flexor muscles. It should be noted that the present tendency is to perform the repair in maximum plantar flexion, in order to reduce the risk of tendon lengthening.

Surgical approach

A postero-medial skin incision is preferred in order to minimize any risk of injury to the sural nerve or its branches. Also, this allows easier access to the plantaris tendon, if needed. In some instances, a longitudinal posterior skin incision is used; however, this may produce a painful scar. The postero-medial incision usually has a length of between 5 and 8 cm. After the paratendon is opened, the frayed tendon ends are easily located, and should be traced proximally and distally to healthy tendon. Very uncommonly, the tendon is avulsed from the calcaneus. The skin and subcutaneous tissues should be handled in an atraumatic fashion to reduce the risk of subsequent soft tissue break-down. After the tendon has been exposed, the gap is cleaned from blood clots, and the tendon ends are freed. Dissection should be kept to a minimum to reduce the risk of further injury. The ends of the tendon are debrided and approximated. This can usually be achieved without major tension. There is much debate about suture selection, and the surgeon's preference plays a role. In most studies, either non-absorbable or absorbable strong core sutures are used. Two parallel strands are commonly used, for example, side-to-side absorbable sutures, with the knots buried in the tendon. However, up to six strands have been used in order to increase the mechanical strength of the repair. The most commonly used suture configurations are Bunnell, Kessler, modified Kessler, and Krackow-types. There are no convincing controlled comparisons between these different suture configurations. In general, a locking-type configuration is preferred, as this increases the mechanical strength of the repair. Other configurations, such wire pull-out are no longer commonly used. It is debatable whether smaller sutures should be placed circumferentially at the tendon repair site to improve the mechanical strength of the repair, and make the repair site smoother. This only increases the tendon repair strength of some 15%, but might increase the risk of vascular compromise.

A three tissue bundle technique has been advocated by many surgeons during the last 30 years. The ruptured tendon is exposed through a standard postero-medial incision avoiding subcutaneous dissection, and to preserve the anterior mesotenon. The disorganized fibres are adapted in three bundles using atraumatic resorbable sutures. With the foot in full equinus, the three bundles are approximated using Bunnell sutures (fig 1.). After closure of the paratenon, the skin is closed with atraumatic sutures. Immediately after the operation, the foot is placed in a plaster cast in a plantigrade position. The strength of the sutures is such that elongation takes place at the muscular level, with no deleterious effect on the sutured tendon.

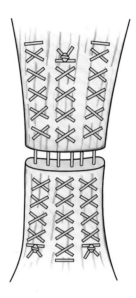

Fig. 1. Triple bundle suture technique

This technique provides a good mechanical strength, and has also been used in neglected ruptures, with a tendon gap up to 4 cm without need for tendon augmentation. A possible disadvantage of the technique is scar tissue formation that causes discomfort in approximately 7-10% of the patients.

Tendon augmentation was traditionally used 20-30 years ago, but it increases the risk of skin healing problems. Augmentation may be considered in case of extreme tissue fraying, when there is a very distal rupture, or a poor holding strength of the sutures. Some surgeons have used artificial ligaments, such as braided polyester and polypropylene, and others have used the plantaris tendon or a proximal section of the Achilles tendon, either as a free flap, or turn-down flap. There are other more complex and accordingly less used possibilities, such as tendon allografts, and transfer of either flexor hallucis longus tendon or peroneal tendons. Augmentation will always require a larger incision and the risk of complications is increased. We do not recommend primary augmentation when performing open repairs of uncomplicated Achilles tendon ruptures[21].

After the repair is completed, the paratenon is carefully sutured, if this can be accomplished without undue tendon, and the skin is sutures using interrupted sutures, although some prefer subcuticular sutures or staples. Post-operatively, the leg is immobilized in a short leg plaster cast or an ankle brace. If the strength of the repair is satisfactory, range of motion exercises are generally started after 10 to14 days, or possibly earlier (immediately) after the repair. After this, weight-bearing with restricted dorsiflexion should be commenced as early as possible.

Prophylaxis for venous thromboembolism (VTE)

Venous thromboembolic complications, such as deep venous thrombosis and pulmonary embolism frequently occur in trauma-patients, often with an asymptomatic course.

Patients with a fracture of the lower extremity or an Achilles tendon rupture, have a risk of DVT of 19%, a risk of proximal DVT of 5%, and symptomatic DVT of 2.7% without prophylaxis[13]. Another study found an incidence of 10% of which only 1% of patients had a symptomatic VTE[7].

Four randomized controlled trials[7,10,11,13] studied prophylaxis with Low Molecular Weight Heparin (LMWH) in patients immobilized in a cast. From these studies, it may be concluded that prophylaxis with LMWH in all patients immobilized in a cast reduces the frequency of asymptomatic DVT; only one study found that LMWH had unsatisfactory effect. This is the reason that in some European countries LMWH is part of standard hospital care. Nevertheless, it is unclear whether this prophylaxis is cost-effective, and whether it prevents clinically relevant VTE. One RCT compared prolonged thromboprophylaxis in patients with Achilles tendon ruptures immobilized in a cast or in a functional brace after surgical treatment. DVT was diagnosed in 16 of 47 patients (34%) in the prophylaxis group, and in 16 of 44 patients (36%) in the placebo group. In conclusion, prophylaxis did not affect the incidence of DVT during immobilization after Achilles tendon rupture surgery[8].

On the basis of these studies, no evidence-based recommendations can be made. Therefore, the clinician can choose whether not to give prophylaxis, to administer it only for the duration of hospital admission, or to continue it until the extremity is fully mobilized. The current consensus, for instance in the Netherlands, is not to administer active VTE prophylaxis in patients undergoing surgery of the lower extremity, or those who have sustained isolated injury to the lower extremity.

Discussion

Direct comparison of different open techniques has rarely been performed. When comparing end-to-end suture with end-to-end suture and augmentation using the plantaris tendon, better surgical outcome concerning local tenderness, skin adhesion, scarring and tendon thickness were seen in the end-to-end suture group[2]. Simple end-to-end suture is safe and reliable, with a low risk of complications compared with plantaris tendon augmentation. On the other hand, Ateschrang and co-workers studied open augmentation repair using the Silfverskiöld technique, with a turn-down flap. In 104 patients, the rerupture rate was 2% and the infection rate 3%[3]. They concluded that the Silfverskiöld augmentation technique was a good alternative, even in high-demand athletes.

Uchiyama and co-workers studied a new technique for surgical Achilles tendon repair designed to allow for more stability and earlier rehabilitation. They operated on 100 patients using the Tsugue suture, where each of five bundles were gathered in a longitudinal direction and secured with a Bunnell-type suture. They concluded that this surgical technique produced strong repair stability, and enabled earlier (2 weeks) weight-bearing and range of motion exercises[20]. Strauss and co-workers studied the post-operative complications after open end-to-end repair of acute Achilles tendon ruptures. Open repair provided consistent good and excellent long-term results[18]. However, the high clinical success rate was associated with relatively high incidence of post-operative complications. Nevertheless, with careful attention to the surgical wound and patient adherence to post-operative rehabilitation protocols, open surgical repair using end-to-end suture is a reliable management option for active patients.

Khan and co-workers performed a meta-analysis of 12 randomised controlled trials, including approximately 800 patients on the effectiveness of different interventions for the management of acute ruptures. They showed that open management of acute Achilles tendon ruptures significantly reduced the risk of rerupture compared with non-surgical management; however, surgical management was associated with significantly higher risk of other complications, such as infections and wound break-down. Surgical risks were reduced by performing percutaneous surgery. Also, post-operative splinting, i.e. the use of functional brace reduced the overall complication rate. In spite of this well-performed meta-analysis there is no overall consensus on the optimal treatment of acute Achilles tendon ruptures.

Conclusions

On the basis of the randomised studies reviewed, there is evidence that open operative management of acute Achilles tendon ruptures significantly reduces the risk of rerupture compared to non-operative management, but has the drawback of a significantly higher risk of other complications, including wound infection.
These complications may be reduced by performing surgery percutaneously, as shown by recent studies. Post-operative splinting in a functional brace rather than a cast appears to reduce hospital stay, time off work and sports, and may lower the overall complication rate[9].
There is inadequate evidence to comment on different suture techniques, different non-operative management regimes, or different aspects of post-operative cast immobilisation.

References

1] Abelseth G, Buckley RE, Pineo GE, Hull R, Rose MS. Incidence of deep-vein thrombosis in patients with fractures of the lower extremity distal to the hip. J Orthop Trauma 1996;10:230-235.
2] Aktas S, Kocaoglu B, Nalnatoglu U, Seyham M, Guven O. End-to-end versus augmented repair on the treatment of Acute Achilles tendon ruptures. J Foot Ankle Surg 2007;46:336-340.
3] Ateschrang A, Gratzer C, Ochs U, Ochs BG, Weise K. Open augmented repair according to Silfverskiöld for Achilles tendon rupture: An alternative for athletes. A Orthop Unfall 2007; 145:207-211.
4] Boele van Hensbroek P, Haverlag R, Ponsen KJ, Levi M, Goslings JC. Tromboseprofylaxe in de traumatologie. Ned Tijdschr Geneeskd 2007;151:234-239 (Article in Dutch).

5] Eriksson BI, Bauer KA, Lassen MR, Turpie AG. Steering committee of the pentasaccharide in hip-fracture surgery study. Fondaparinux compared with Enoxaparin for the prevention of venous thromboembolism after hip-fracture surgery. N Engl J Med 2001;345:1298-1304.

6] Jaakola JI, Hutton WC, Beskin JL, Lee GP. Achilles tendon rupture repair: Biomechanical comparison of the triple bundle technique versus the Krakow locking loop technique. Foot Ankle Int 2000;21:14-17.

7] Jorgensen PS, Warming T, Hansen K, Paltved C, Vibeke Berg H, Jensen R, Kirchhoff- Jensen R, Kjaer L, Kerbouche N, Leth-Espensen P, Narvestad E, Rasmussen SW, Sloth C, Torholm C, Wille-Jorgensen P. Low molecular weight heparin (Innohep) as tromboprophylaxis in outpatients with a plaster cast: a venografic controlled study. Thromb Res 2002;105:477-480.

8] Kerkhoffs GM, Struijs PA, Raaymakers EL, Marti RK. Functional treatment after surgical repair of acute Achilles tendon rupture: wrap vs walking cast. Arch Orthop Trauma Surg 2002;122:102-105.

9] Khan RJ, Fick D, Keogh A, Crawford J, Brammar T, Parker M. Treatment of acute Achilles tendon ruptures. A meta-analysis of randomized, controlled trials. J Bone Joint Surg 2006; 88-A:1160-1168.

10] Kock H, Schmit-Neuerburg KP, Hanke J, Rudofsky G, Hirche H. Thromboprophylaxis with low-molecular-weight heparin in outpatients with plaster cast immobilisation of the leg. Lancet 1995;346:459-461.

11] Kujath P, Spannagel U, Habscheid W. Incidence and prophylaxis of deep venous thrombosis in outpatients with injury of the lower limb. Haemost 1993;21(Suppl 1):20-26.

12] Lapidus LJ, Rosfors S, Ponzer S, Levander C, Elvin A, Lärfars G, de Bri E.
Prolonged thromboprophylaxis with dalteparin after surgical treatment of Achilles tendon rupture: a randomized, placebo-controlled study. J Orthop Trauma 2007;21:52-57.

13] Lassen MR, Borris LC, Nakov RL. Use of the low-molecular-weight heparin reviparin to prevent deep-vein thrombosis after leg injury requiring immobilization. N Engl J Med 2002;347:726-730.

14] Lo IK, Kirkley A, Nonweiler B, Kumbhare DA. Operative versus non-operative treatment of acute Achilles tendon ruptures: A quantitative review. Clin J Sports Med 1997;3:207-211.

15] Maffulli N, Tallon C, Wong J, Lim KP, Bleakney R. Early weight-bearing and ankle mobilization after open repair of acute midsubstance tears of the Achilles tendon. Am J Sports Med 2003;31:692-700.

16] Park HG, Moon DH, Yoon JM. Limited open repair of ruptured Achilles tendons with Bunnel-type sutures. Foot Ankle Int 2001;22:985-987.

17] Richardsson LC, Reitman R, Wilson M. Achilles tendon ruptures: Functional outcome of surgical repair with a "pull-out" wire. Foot Ankle Int 2003;24:439-443.

18] Strauss EJ, Ishak C, Jazrawi L, Sherman O, Rosen J. Operative treatment of acute Achilles tendon ruptures: An institutional review of clinical outcomes. Injury 2007;38:822-828.

19] Tallon C, Maffulli N, Ewen SW. Ruptured Achilles tendons are significantly more degenerated than tendinopathic tendons. Med Sci Sports Exerc 2001;33:1983-1990.

20] Uchiyama E, Nomura A, Takeda Y, Hiranuma K, Iwaso H. A modified operation for Achilles tendon ruptures. Am J Sports Med 2007;ePub.

21] CBO Dutch Guideline for Diagnostics, Prevention, and Treatment of Venous Thrombo Embolism and Secondary Prevention of Arterial Thrombosis, Dutch Institute for Health Care Improvement 2008 (in Dutch).

"Small is beautiful"

(E. F. Schumacher)

Chapter 7.

MINIMALLY INVASIVE AND PERCUTANEOUS SURGERY

Robin R. Elliot, James D. F. Calder

Take Home Message

• *Modern techniques combine the benefits of visualizing tendon apposition at the rupture site with percutaneous methods.*
• *Knowledge of the anatomy of the sural nerve is essential.*
• *Consider early functional rehabilitation.*

Introduction

There remains no consensus opinion regarding the gold standard treatment of acute rupture of the Achilles tendon. If the clinician and patient opt for surgery, there is further debate regarding which of the recognized surgical procedures produces the best outcome.

Conservative treatment may lead to problems associated with re-rupture, lengthening of the tendon and poor function, whereas surgery introduces additional risks of wound breakdown, infection, scar adhesions and sural nerve damage.

Percutaneous and mini-open surgical repair techniques were developed in order to minimize the potential risks of surgery and to improve functional outcomes. In general these techniques have met their stated goals, but that has not always been the case as will be explained in this overview.

Basic science

The pathology underpinning the mechanism of failure of the Achilles tendon is still not fully understood, but some of the intrinsic characteristics of tendons, namely hypovascularity and hypocellularity, may explain its slow rate of healing. Tendon healing occurs through described phases: inflammation, proliferation, repair, and remodeling. During the healing process, tendons respond to stress in a similar manner to bones: they remodel, becoming stronger and stiffer. This is achieved by an increase in collagen synthesis and alteration in fibre alignment. For this reason, movement is now widely believed to be an important component of the post-operative rehabilitation regime.

Suture material strongly influences the biomechanical performance of multistrand tendon repairs and is an important consideration for the surgeon[13].

Treatment Techniques

Although open surgical repair was described as early as the tenth century AD[4], Ma and Griffiths were the first to describe a percutaneous repair technique for the acute Achilles rupture[14]. Their construct incorporates a Bunnell suture through the proximal stump and a box suture through the distal stump (Figure 1). The sutures are passed via six stab incisions, three on either side of the tendon.

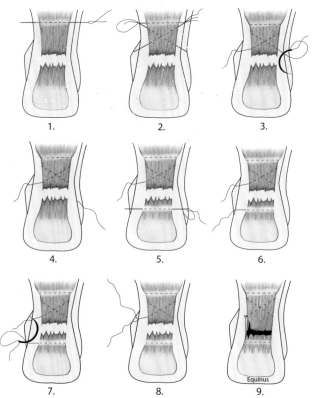

Figure 1. Ma and Griffiths´ technique for percutaneous repair of acute ruptured Achilles tendon.

58

This technique has been modified to improve gapping resistance at the repair site by using more passes of the suture material through the distal stump[7,9]. A two-cohort study (237 patients) comparing this modified percutaneous technique to a standard open repair found equivalent functional outcomes in both groups, but less overall complications in the percutaneous group[8].

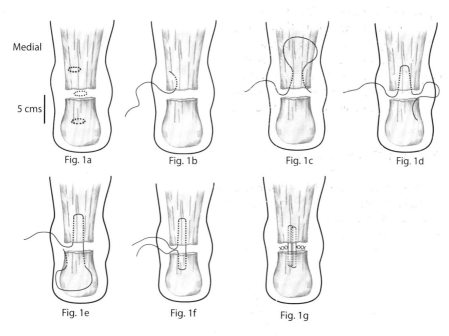

Medial

5 cms

Fig. 1a   Fig. 1b   Fig. 1c   Fig. 1d

Fig. 1e   Fig. 1f   Fig. 1g

Figure 2: Webb and Bannister technique
Diagrams showing 1a) the position of the three skin incisions, 1b) the suture entering the middle incision, passing through the tendon and out of the proximal incision, 1c) the suture re-entering the proximal incision, back through the tendon and exiting from the middle incision, 1d) again entering the middle incision, passing through the distal tendon and out of the distal incision, 1e) capturing of the distal tendon stump, 1f) completion of the box stitch and 1g) the placing of a second suture in the tendon before tying both sutures.

Webb and Bannister developed their percutaneous technique with the specific aim of reducing the incidence of sural nerve injury, which seemed to be at significant risk when performing percutaneous repairs[22]. Their technique uses only three skin incisions, which are placed away from the lateral side of the tendon in order to protect the sural nerve (figure 2). A similar technique has been described by McClelland and Maffulli[18].
The Tenolig® device (Fournitures Hospitalieres Industrie, France) is a percutaneous technique which uses a harpoon device (Figure 3), however, a case series of

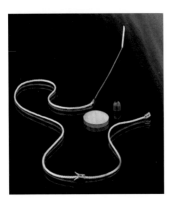

Figure 3: 'Harpoon tenorrhaphy'
Two stab incision are made 4-5cm proximal to the rupture. The harpoon is passed through the proximal stump, the rupture site and the distal stump by palpation, exiting through the skin either side of the calcaneus. The construct is tensioned through barbs proximally and lead crimps distally. The wire is removed after 6 weeks.

124 patients treated using this device reported significant complications including suture and device failure and a high rate of re-rupture (10%) and sural nerve entrapment (5.2%)[15].

A cadaveric study[9] revealed malaligned stumps in four of five tendons repaired with the Ma and Griffiths' technique. However, the clinical significance of the malalignment is unclear, as, in clinical practice, results of the Ma and Griffiths' technique is acceptable.

A number of surgeons have made efforts to devise mini-open approaches to Achilles tendon repair. Such techniques have certain advantages, as one can see the rupture site, remove interposed tissue, and see whether appropriate tendon stump juxtaposition has been achieved[2,11,20].

Kakiuchi reported on a technique that employed a combined percutaneous and limited open repair[11]. The gap in the tendon is palpated and a small incision is made at this level, allowing the tendon stumps to be identified. A repair is then performed percutaneously, assisted by the use of two crude suture passing devices, fashioned from bent 2 mm Kirschner wires, which are passed beneath the paratenon (Figure 4). This technique ensures good tendon apposition and the sutures are placed well away from the diseased area of tendon.

The principles of Kakiuchi's technique together with information obtained from a cadaveric study led to the development of a guiding instrument to perform this type of repair2. This instrument is now marketed as a single-use, rigid polymer device called Achillon (Integra Lifesciences Corporation, USA) which has a shape (8° V angle) and cross-sectional area (81mm²) based upon the anatomy of the tendons of the cadaveric specimens (Figure 5).

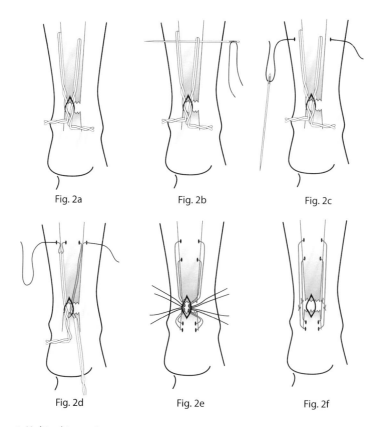

Fig. 2a Fig. 2b Fig. 2c

Fig. 2d Fig. 2e Fig. 2f

Figure 4: Kakiuchi repair

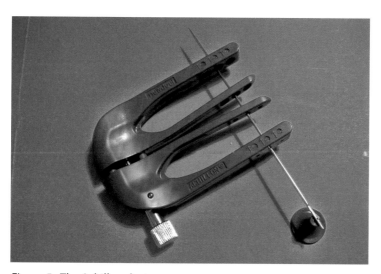

Figure 5: The Achillon device

The Achillon system combines the percutaneous passage of the sutures with the benefit of visual control at the repair site. The likelihood of sural nerve entrapment is reduced because the sutures are retrieved by the inner arms of the device which are placed beneath the paratenon layer. A single incision is made at the level of the rupture and the procedure can be performed under local anesthetic (Figure 6).

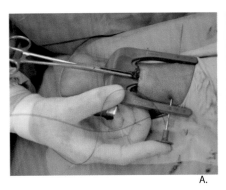 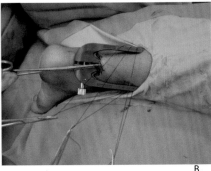

A. B.

Figure 6: (A) Passing suture (B) Sutures in situ prior to removal of introducer

Tips and tricks

Identification of the correct level for skin incision is important to visualize the apposition of the tendon ends as the sutures are tied. Although a longitudinal incision was originally described, a horizontal incision leads to better healing and a more cosmetically acceptable scar. The optimal placement of this incision appears to be 1 cm distal to the palpable proximal stump, allowing the proximal end to be drawn down under tension and the distal stump to be brought up to the wound level by plantar flexion of the ankle.

The Achillon device is made of plastic and care must be taken to ensure that the arms do not twist or bend as this can lead to the suture needle missing the guide hole. Finally all sutures should be tested individually to ensure that they have a good hold in the tendon and are individually capable of drawing the tendon stump to the level of the wound.

Short-term after treatment

Traditionally, acutely repaired Achilles tendon ruptures have been treated postoperatively in a plaster cast, which is serially altered to bring the foot to a plantigrade position over approximately six weeks. This may lead to calf muscle atrophy, joint stiffness, adhesion formation and an increased risk of deep vein thrombosis. In recent times, more functional rehabilitation regimes have gained popularity[6].

Studies have shown that early functional rehabilitation can increase the strength of healed tendons[14] and shorten rehabilitation time16. Percutaneous and mini-open techniques reduce problems with wound healing and therefore may be most suited to early mobilization.

Our patients are given a functional ankle orthotic device, applied in theatre at the time of surgery. The foot is positioned at 20° plantarflexion during wound healing, as this is the optimal position for skin perfusion[21]. Early weight bearing is encouraged, and, from two weeks, free plantarflexion, limiting dorsiflexion past plantigrade. Physiotherapy is commenced at two weeks.

Complications (and how to reduce them)

Infection

Infection is significantly reduced when comparing percutaneous and open surgical techniques (0% vs 19.6%)[12]. Any surgical procedure should be undertaken with care in patients with diabetes or vascular disease, smokers, and those taking corticosteroids. However, it could be argued that these patients would benefit even more from a minimally invasive approach. The surgeon must handle the soft tissues carefully. A tourniquet is not required for mini-open and percutaneous repair.

Rerupture

A recent meta-analysis has shown rerupture to be reduced threefold with operative techniques with less rerupture in the percutaneous pooled group (2.1% vs 4.3%). Post-operative functional bracing with early weight bearing and mobilization may lead to a stronger repair and less rerupture.

Sural nerve damage

A sound knowledge of the anatomy of the sural nerve and care taken when passing sutures should help to prevent damage to this structure. Anatomical studies have shown a significant degree of variability in the location of the sural nerve in relation to the Achilles tendon[1,22], which can complicate attempts to avoid entrapment. Exposure of the nerve through extended incisions[17] and use of the Achillon device[2] have been shown to reduce the incidence of nerve injury.

Adhesion Formation

There is less concern in terms of wound healing when using mini-open and percutaneous methods. For this reason, mobilization can be started early in the post-operative period. This early motion at the repair site combined with a less invasive repair reduces the chance of troublesome adhesions forming. There is no conclusive evidence yet that the use of hyaluronate preparations reduces adhesions.

Outcome

The lack of well conducted studies into the outcomes after Achilles rupture and the efficacy of different treatment modalities is highlighted by the two main meta-analyses on this subject[12,24]. Maffulli and co-workers showed that study methodology has improved over time, however Khan and co-workers found only 12 studies that were worthy of inclusion in their meta-analysis. They showed a pooled rate of rerupture was 4.3% (two of forty-six) in the open group and 2.1% (one of forty-eight) in the percutaneous group (relative risk, 2.00; 95% confidence interval, 0.19 to 21.00). Percutaneous repair was associated with a lower complication rate (excluding rerupture) compared with open operative repair (relative risk, 2.84; 95% confidence interval, 1.06 to 7.62). Patients who had been managed with a functional brace postoperatively (allowing for early mobilization) had a lower complication rate compared with those who had been managed with a cast (relative risk, 1.88; 95% confidence interval, 1.27 to 2.76).

Assal and co-workers reported by on a consecutive series of 87 patients managed using the Achillon device[2]. The results revealed good AOFAS scores (mean 96 points) at an average 26 month follow up, with no significant difference between the injured and uninjured sides on isokinetic and endurance testing: all patients returned to previous levels of sporting activity. In addition, there were no cases of wound infections or sural nerve disturbance. Calder and Saxby replicated these favorable results in a review of 46 patients treated with this technique[3].

Ceccarelli and co-workers compared the modified Ma and Griffith repair with the Achillon system in a prospective two cohort study where post-operatively both groups were treated with the same semi-functional rehabilitation regime using a walker boot[5]. The two groups were equivalent in terms of complications (no infections, no re-ruptures, no sural nerve injuries), AOFAS scores and return to sports activity.

In vitro studies have examined the strength of the Achillon repair[10]. Ismail and co-workers studied matched groups of sheep Achilles tendons that were repaired, using either the Achillon or a Kessler suture, and tested for mean load to failure. The Achillon was found to be a mechanically sound method of repair with comparable tensile strength to a Kessler repair (153 N ±60 versus 123 N ±24). It should be noted, however, that the Achillon suture used a total of six strands of suture material versus four strands used in the Kessler repair.

Conclusion

Surgical techniques for treating acute Achilles rupture are changing and there appears to be an increasing role for percutaneous and mini-open techniques. Some studies suggest that these techniques can give results equivalent to or better than those of an open repair, with the added benefit of fewer complications. Evidence suggests that early functional rehabilitation can increase the strength of healed tendons and shorten rehabilitation time; early mobilization may be allowed in patients treated with these methods. Further well conducted, prospective, randomized studies are needed to settle the debate over the best treatment for the acute rupture of the Achilles tendon, however a combined minimally invasive/percutaneous technique with early functional rehabilitation would seem to be the current gold standard.

References

1] Aktan Ikiz I, Ucerler H, Bilge O. The anatomic features of the sural nerve with an emphasis on its clinical importance. Foot Ankle Int 2005;26:560-567.

2] Assal M, Jung M, Stern R et al. Limited open repair of Achilles tendon ruptures: a technique with a new instrument and findings of a prospective multi-center study. J Bone Joint Surg Am 2002;84:161-170.

3] Calder JD, Saxby TS. Early, active rehabilitation following mini-open repair of Achilles tendon rupture: a prospective study. Br J Spots Med 2005;39:857-859.

4] Carlstedt CA. Mechanical and chemical factors in tendon healing. Effects of indomethacin and surgery in the rabbit. Acta Orthop Scand, Suppl 1987; 224.

5] Ceccarelli F, Berti L, Giuriati L et al. Percutaneous and minimally invasive techniques of Achilles tendon repair. Clin Orthop Relat Res 2007 [Epub ahead of print].

6] Cetti R, Henriksen LO, Jacobsen KS. A new treatment of ruptured Achilles tendons. A prospective randomized study. Clin Orthop Relat Res 1994;308:155-165.

7] Cretnik A, Zlapjpah L, Smrkolj V et al. The strength of percutaneous methods of repair of the Achilles tendon: a biomechanical study. Med Sci Sports Exerc 2000;32:16-20.

8] Cretnik A, Kasanovic M, Smrkolj V. Percutaneous versus open repair of the ruptured Achilles tendon: a comparative study. Am J Sports Med 2005;33:1369-79.

9] Hockenbury R, Johns J. A biomechanical in vitro comparison of open versus percutaneous repair of tendon Achilles. Foot Ankle 1990;11:67-72.

10] Ismail M, Karim A, Calder J. The Achillon achilles tendon repair - is it strong enough? [Abstract] EFFORT Congress 2007.

11] Kakiuchi M. A combined open and percutaneous technique for repair of tendo Achillis: Comparison with open repair. J Bone Joint Surg Br1995;77:60-63.

12] Khan R, Fick D, Keogh A et al. Treatment of Acute Achilles Tendon Ruptures. A Meta-Analysis of Randomized, Controlled Trials. J Bone Joint Surg Am 2005;87:2202 -2210.

13] Lawrence TM, Davis RC. A biomechanical analysis of suture materials and their influence on a four-strand flexor tendon repair. J Hand Surg 2005;30: 836-841.

14] Ma GWC, Griffith TG. Percutaneous repair of acute closed ruptured Achilles tendon: a new technique. Clin Orthop 1977;128:247-255.

15] Maes R, Copin G, Averous C. Is percutaneous repair of the Achilles tendon a safe technique? A study of 124 cases. Acta Orthop Belg 2006;72:179-183.

16] Maffulli N, Tallon C, Wong J et al. Early weightbearing and ankle mobilization after open repair of acute midsubstance tears of the achilles tendon. Am J Sports Med 2003;31:692-700.

17] Majewski M, Rohrbach M, Czaja S et al. Avoiding sural nerve injuries during percutaneous Achilles tendon repair. Am J Sports Med 2006;34:793-798.

18] McClelland D, Maffulli N. Percutaneous repair of ruptured Achilles tendon. Journal of the Royal College of Surgeons of Edinburgh 2002;41:613–618.

19] Palmes D, Spiegel H, Schneider T et al. Achilles tendon healing: long-term biomechanical effects of postoperative mobilization and immobilization in a new mouse model. J Orthop Res 2002;20:939-946.

20] Park H, Moon D, Yoon J. Limited open repair of ruptured Achilles tendons with Bunnel-type sutures. Foot Ankle Int 2001;22:985-987.

21] Poynton A, O'Rourke K. An analysis of skin perfusion over the achilles tendon in varying degrees of plantarflexion. Foot Ankle Int 2001;22:572-574.

22] Webb JM, Bannister GC. Percutaneous repair of the ruptured tendo Achillis. J Bone Joint Surg Br 1999;81:877-880.

23] Webb J, Moorjani N, Radford M. Anatomy of the sural nerve and its relation to the Achilles tendon. Foot Ankle Int 2000;21:475-477.

24] Wong J, Barrass V, Maffulli N. Quantitative review of operative and nonoperative management of Achilles tendon ruptures. Am J Sports Med 2002;30:565-575.

"Come then, let us go forward together with our united strength."

(Winston Churchill)

Chapter 8.

MECHANICAL TESTING OF DIFFERENT SUTURE TECHNIQUES

Michael J. Lutz, James D.F. Calder

Take Home Message

• *A triple bundle or Krackow locking loop technique provide the strongest repairs. Incorporating a bone tunnel for suture passage or using bone anchors does not significantly increase the load to failure.*
• *A Polyblend suture has a significantly higher ultimate load and leads to significantly smaller gap formation.*
• *The preferred suture size for the majority of mechanical tests of Achilles tendon repairs has been Number 1 and 2 sutures.*
• *Experimental studies have shown that repetitive cyclic loading leads to gap formation, the size of the gap being the smallest in Polyblend sutured tendons.*
• *We recommend that in case of functional after-treatment repairs be performed with "overtightened" tension or apparent tendon shortening to allow for the impending lengthening that will occur during rehabilitation.*

Introduction

Surgical management of Achilles tendon ruptures should provide better functional outcome than non-operative management. This is achieved if patients have shorter rehabilitation times and improved short- and/or long-term function, without exposure to an unacceptable risk of complications. The ability of suture techniques to resist re-rupture and repair gap formation has an integral role in this balance.

Multiple suture techniques have been described. These include the Kessler, modifications of Kessler, Bunnel, Krackow Locking-loop, Triple Bundle, Boxed Loop, Ma-Griffith and techniques which include bone anchors or tunnels. Mechanical testing of these techniques has addressed the ultimate loads to failure, the effect of different suture materials, the effect of repetitive cycling, the modes of failure, the effect of tendon morphology and the post-operative strength of the affected gastrocnemius-soleus musculotendinous complex.

Suture Technique

Testing the ultimate load to failure has been performed using servo-hydraulic tensile testing devices[1,2,3,4,5,6,7,8,9]. The load at which gap formation appears is also frequently recorded. Resistance to failure and gap formation is increased by increasing the number of transverse passes across the tendon, increasing the number of suture strands crossing the rupture site and increasing the number of locking passes[1,2,3,4,5,6,7,8,10]. Incorporating a bone tunnel for suture passage or using bone anchors does not significantly increase the load to failure[9]. Therefore, either a Triple Bundle or Krackow Locking Loop technique provide the strongest repairs. The superiority of these techniques is reinforced by the results of "Modes of Failure" and "Tendon Morphology".

The modes of failure seen in testing models have been recorded. Techniques with combined transverse and locking loops fail within the suture or at the knot. The techniques without locking loops, e.g. Boxed Loop, fail either within the suture or by suture cut-out[6]. Bone anchor techniques failed by anchor pull-out[9].

The effect of tendon morphology on the mechanical strength of Achilles tendon suture techniques has also been assessed. The Boxed Loop technique, which does not have locking passes, is less resistant in narrower tendons. These sutures are prone to cutting out of the narrower tendons, and it may reflect the decreased transverse purchase in the tendon[6].

Figure 1. Suture Techniques

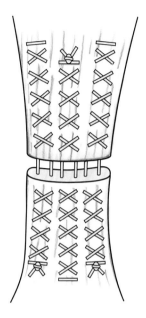

1a. Triple Bundle

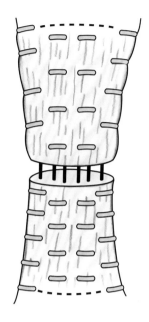

1b. Krakow Locking Loop

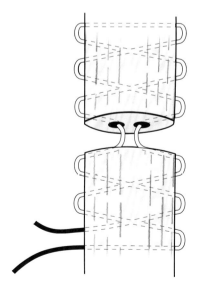

1c. Bunnel

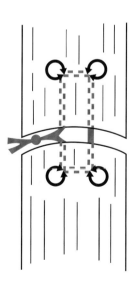

1d. Kessler

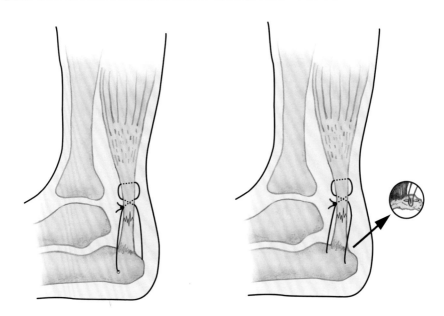

1e. Calcaneal Tunnel and Bone Anchor

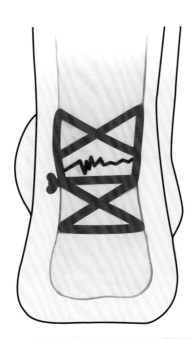

1f. Ma - Griffith Percutaneous Technique

Suture Material and Size

The load to failure and the load to gap formation are also influenced by the type of suture used. Polyester sutures have been the most commonly used suture in mechanical tests[3,5,6,7,8,9]. Few comparative studies have been performed but results indicate that non-absorbable Polyester (Ti-cron™ and Ethibond™) sutures are more resistant to failure than absorbable braided and monofilament options (PDS II™, Panacryl™, Vicryl™ and Silk)[1,3,4,5,6,7,8,9]. Polyester sutures also demonstrate superior knot security[3].

Despite the prevalence of Polyester in mechanical tests, recent studies have demonstrated that non-absorbable Polyblend (polyethylene core with braided polyester coating) suture (Fibrewire™) outperforms non-absorbable Polyester suture (Ethibond™)[2,11]. The Polyblend suture has a significantly higher ultimate load and significantly smaller gap formation[2].

In Achilles tendon models, there are no known direct comparisons of any one suture material in varying diameters. There is no mechanical testing evidence to confirm that a larger diameter number 2 polyester suture is more resistant to failure than a number 0 polyester suture. However, the preferred suture sizes for the majority of mechanical tests of Achilles tendon repairs have been Numbers 1 and 2[1,2,3,4,6,7,8,9].

Early Rehabilitation

Early active functional rehabilitation is common following operative Achilles tendon repair. Repetitive cycling mechanical models have been used to replicate this clinical scenario. In these tests, servo-hydraulic tensile devices are used to repeatedly apply and then release a constant force across the repair[2]. This is opposed to the ultimate load tests, which gradually increase the distraction force until failure occurs.

In a repetitive cycling test comparing number 2 Polyblend and number 2 Polyester sutures used in a Krackow Locking Loop technique, there were no failures of either suture due to cycling with loads up to 125N for 3000 cycles. However, gap formation was noted. The size of the gap was significantly smaller for the Polyblend repaired tendon. For both types of suture material, the size of the gap increased with the number of cycles performed[2].

Gap formation equates to a lengthened, mechanically disadvantaged repair that has delayed accrual of repair-site strength[5]. If early rehabilitation is adopted for post-operative care, allowance for this phenomenon should be incorporated into the repair technique.

Shortcomings of the Current Experimental Models

There are some obvious limitations that must be acknowledged for all forms of Achilles suture technique mechanical testing. Foremost is the inability to replicate the clinical tendon rupture pattern in vitro. To date, in vitro mechanical tests have assessed suture technique for transversely sectioned, healthy tendons and not the oedematous, frayed "Horse Hair" or "Mop End" tendons present in the clinical scenario. The effect of this difference has not and, probably, may not be evaluated.

In vitro mechanical testing also does not account for the effect that each suture technique has on tendon vascularity and therefore healing capabilities. It may be that the strongest suture techniques result in tissue "strangulation" and therefore counteract the positive effect of the particular technique.

Another limitation is that some studies have assessed suture techniques in animal models. All other studies have used human cadaveric tissue. Micro- and macroscopic differences with in vivo tissue may be clinically and biologically significant.

The absence of a recognised "Gold Standard" or "Control" suture technique has resulted in numerous comparative studies which are difficult to interpret beyond the direct comparisons tested in each individual study. Similarly, whilst we can extrapolate that a suture technique is mechanically sound based on its clinical results, no minimum or baseline mechanical testing standards or values have been established.

Conclusion and Recommendations

Mechanical testing has provided a number of useful facts that can be transferred into the clinical field. Based on current biomechanical evidence, we recommend achieving the strongest possible repair, most resistance to failure and gap formation by utilising a Number 1 or 2 Polyblend (Fibrewire™) suture in a Krackow Locking Loop or Triple Bundle Technique. The suitability of this biomechanically optimal repair should be balanced by clinical factors and risks associated with wound exposure, the effect on tendon vascularity and the proximity of the sural nerve.

Mechanical tests have also demonstrated that gap formation appears inevitable with all current Achilles tendon suture techniques. A concluding recommendation would be that, in case of functional after-treatment, repairs should be performed with "overtightened" tension or apparent tendon shortening to allow for the impending lengthening that will occur during rehabilitation.

Tissue	Technique	Suture Material	No. of strands	Load to failure (N)	Author
Human	Kessler	1 Ethibond	2	85	Watson *et al*
Human	Bunnell	1 Ethibond	2	93	Watson *et al*
Human	Ma-Griffith	2 Vicryl	1	111	Cretnik *et al*
Ovine	Kessler	2 Ticron	2	123	Ismail *et al*
Human	Krackow Locking Loop	1 Ethibond	4	147	Watson *et al*
Ovine	Boxed Loop	2 Ticron	6	153	Ismail *et al*
Human	Double Kessler	1-0 Silk	4	154	Gerdes *et al*
Human	Krackow Locking Loop	1 Ethibond	4	161	Jaakkola *et al*
Human	Bone Anchor	1 Panacryl	4	166	Zandbergen *et al*
Human	Bone Anchor	1 PDS-II	4	185	Zandbergen *et al*
Human	Calcaneal Tunnel	1 Panacryl	4	186	Zandbergen *et al*
Human	Calcaneal Tunnel	1 PDS-II	4	195	Zandbergen *et al*
Human	Bunnell	1 PDS-II	2	211	Zandbergen *et al*
Human	Modified Ma-Griffith	2 Vicryl	1	214	Cretnik *et al*
Human	Double Kessler with Flap	1-0 Silk	4	218	Gerdes *et al*

Bovine	Krackow Locking Loop	2 Ethibond	4	222	Benthien *et al*
Human	Triple Bundle	1 Ethibond	6	453	Jaakkola *et al*
Bovine	Krackow Locking Loop	2 Fibrewire	4	582	Benthien *et al*

Table 1: Ultimate Loads to Failure of Cadaveric Achilles Tendon Mechanical Tests

References

1] Assal M, Jung M, Stern R, Rippstein P, Delmi M, Hoffmeyer P. Limited open repair of Achilles tendon ruptures: a technique with a new instrument and findings of a prospective multicenter study. J Bone Joint Surg 2002;84-A:161-70.

2] Benthien R, Aronow M, Doran-Diaz V, Sullivan R, Naujoks R, Adams D. Cyclic Loading of Achilles Tendon Repairs: A Comparison of Polyester and Polyblend Suture. Foot Ankle Int 2006;27:512-518.

3] Bibbo C, Milia M, Gehrmann R, Patel D, Anderson R. Strength and Knot Security of Braided Polyester and Caprolactone/Glycolide Suture. Foot Ankle Int 2004;24:712-715.

4] Cretnik A, Zlajpah L, Smrkolj V, Kosanovic M. The strength of percutaneous methods of repair of the Achilles tendon: a biomechanical study. Med Sci Sports Exerc 2000;32:16-20.

5] Gerdes MH, Brown TD, Bell AL, Baker JA, Levson M, Layer S. A flap augmentation technique for Achilles tendon repair. Postoperative strength and functional outcome. Clin Orthop Relat Res 1992;280:241-246.

6] Ismail M, Karim A, Amis A, Calder J. The Achillon Achilles Tendon Repair – Is it strong enough? Accepted for publication Foot Ankle Int 2007.

7] Jaakkola JI, Hutton WC, Beskin JL, Lee GP. Achilles tendon rupture repair: biomechanical comparison of the triple bundle technique versus the Krakow locking loop technique. Foot Ankle Int 2000;21:14-17.

8] Watson TW, Jurist KA, Yang KH, Shen KL. The strength of Achilles tendon repair: an in vitro study of the biomechanical behaviour in human cadaver tendons. Foot Ankle Int 1995;16:191-195.

9] Zandbergen RA, de Boer SF, Swierstra BA, Day J, Kleinrensink GJ, Beumer A. Surgical treatment of Achilles tendon rupture: examination of strength of 3 types of suture techniques in a cadaver model. Acta Orthop 2005;76:408-411.

10] Silva MJ, Boyer MI, Gelberman RH: Recent progress in flexor tendon healing. J Orthop Sci 2002;7:508-514.

11] Acton D, Perry A, Evans R, Butler A, Stephens P, Bruce W, Goldberg J, Sonna bend D, Walsh W. The effect of two nonresorbable suture types on the mechanical performance over a metal suture anchor eyelet. Knee Surgery Sports Traumatology Arthroscopy 2004;12:165-168.

Chapter 9.

CONSERVATIVE TREATMENT

Richard G.H. Wallace

Take home message

• *Conservative management of acute AT rupture can be effective in all age groups and for both sedentary and sporting individuals.*
• *Conservative management must be supervised by a senior and experienced surgeon. It requires much commitment, and is not an easy alternative to surgery.*
• *Dynamic mobilisation during the second month of management with protection of the healing tendon with an appropriate orthosis is an essential step of management.*

Background

The best management for acute Achilles tendon (AT) rupture is still hotly debated. Those supporting the surgical approach feel that the correct tendon tension can only be achieved by direct visualisation, and further suggest that surgical repair results in a lower rerupture[1,2,3,4]. Also, open repair is said to allow earlier ankle mobilisation. However, surgery involves hospital admission, anaesthesia, wound healing problems, and increased cost.
Most publications on the management of Achilles tendon rupture refer to surgical management, and generally deal with relatively small numbers of patients[5,7,9]. There have been only a few prospective randomised studies, and in most stud-

ies classical immobilisation in plaster cast has been used, rather than functional bracing[5,8,9]. Functional bracing for the management of acute Achilles tendon tears was developed by McComis and co-workers [7], but again the numbers were small.

Non-surgical management of Achilles tendon rupture is not a new concept. John Hunter ruptured his Achilles tendon while dancing and treated himself with strapping. Pels-Leusden advocated this method in the early 1900's[10].

Elderly, medically unfit patients with acute Achilles tendon rupture managed conservatively can do well, although this is not supported by large cohort studies. Hence, if older individuals who could be expected to have poorer healing still recovered well without surgery, then younger and fitter patients might be expected to do at least as well.

Furthermore, when operated on within 24 hours of rupture, as the Achilles tendon was exposed, with the ankle well plantar flexed and prior to any clearance of haematoma, the tendon ends came together anatomically without further assistance. Attempts to suture two ragged tendon ends inevitably leads to some bunching up of the tendon. The suture, far from imparting any functional strength, simply holds the tendon ends in good anatomical position while natural healing and repair takes place. If this could be achieved reliably by conservative means, then surgical intervention would surely not be required.

A protocol for conservative management of acute Achilles tendon rupture has therefore been developed. Only those patients who had been placed in an equinus cast within 24 hours of rupture were included in the initial trial. The equinus position was maintained in a cast for four weeks with the patient strictly non-weight bearing. A removable custom made orthosis was then provided with overshoe and weight-bearing commenced. Patients used this orthosis for four weeks. They were advised to remove the orthosis in bed at night and also during the day while seated to perform regular active ankle exercises.

After 140 patients had been managed successfully using this protocol, the protocol was changed and the custom-made orthosis changed to a pneumatic walker including appropriate heel raises within the splint to improve convenience and comfort. The rocker sole of the brace further protects the healing tendon by reducing the lever effect of the foot during walking. At an early stage in the development of the management protocol structured physiotherapy was introduced with good effect.

A preliminary study of the first 32 consecutive patients presenting with acute Achilles tendon rupture was encouraging[9], which led to further work, in which an independent physiotherapist carried out a detailed study of the next 140 consecutive patients[11]. I have now personally treated over 1,000 consecutive patients using the conservative protocol. The re-rupture rate is less than 4%. All those suffering a re-rupture were again treated using the same conservative regime with excellent results in all but three who required surgery after which they did well. One patient, an orthopaedic surgeon, who sustained an early complete rerupture, was able to return to highly competitive international tennis following a second course of conservative management. Many patients treated conservatively have returned to their previous sporting activities.

Protocol

Patients presenting at A&E departments with suspected acute Achilles tendon rupture are placed in an equinus plaster of Paris cast and referred to a weekly central Achilles tendon rupture clinic. Ideally they will be seen at this clinic between one and two weeks after the rupture. The cast is removed and the patient is assessed.

Observation of the patient with a recent Achilles tendon rupture will reveal classical bruising on both medial and lateral sides of the heel (Figures 1 a & b). This bruised area will not be tender and there will be no bony tenderness about the ankle.

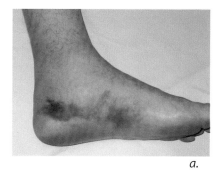 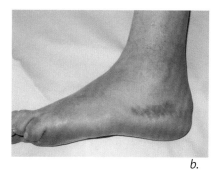

a. *b.*

Fig. 1: Bruising on medial (a) and lateral (b) sides of the heel

A calf muscle tear is excluded and the tendon itself is examined. With tenderness over the Achilles tendon and a palpable gap one can be confident of the diagnosis. The absence of plantar flexion on calf squeeze adds further reassurance to this diagnosis.

The ankle is then plantar flexed, and the tendon palpated to ensure that the tendon ends are felt to oppose well. This is a reliable clinical test in experienced hands and it rare that further tests such as ultrasound will be required. A suitably padded synthetic cast is applied with sufficient plantar flexion to achieve satisfactory apposition of the tendon ends (Fig. 2). The patient is then instructed to remain strictly non-weight bearing until their next appointment at the clinic. The conservative management of the rupture, expected progress and outcome are all explained in appropriate detail to the patient and those accompanying them. Protection in a plantar flexed cast continues for a total of four weeks from the date of rupture. Patients remain strictly non-weight-bearing all this time.

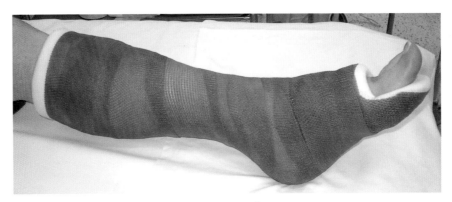

Fig. 2: padded synthetic cast applied in plantar flexion

The cast is then removed, and the integrity of the Achilles tendon is assessed by an experienced clinician. The tendon is first palpated to ensure continuity. The patient is then asked actively to plantar flex the foot against resistance of a single finger of the examiner whilst the examiner's other hand palpates the tendon, feeling for any "fibre tearing". The examiner gradually applies an increasing resistance while still palpating the tendon. By this means it is possible to ascertain if the tendon has healed sufficiently to progress to the next stage of the treatment. If not, a further week or two in equinus cast may occasionally be required – such as in a rheumatoid patient on steroids.

Where the healing progress is considered satisfactory a pneumatic walker of suitable size is fitted. Heel raises are added to allow comfortable weight bearing on the heel. The height of the raise varies from one patient to another.

The pneumatic walker is to be worn at all times when standing or walking for four weeks. It is stressed that standing or trying to hop without the brace is absolutely forbidden. Patients are advised that they may weight bear fully in this brace, but usually require the support of crutches for the first day or two. The splint may be removed in bed with strict instructions that it must be reapplied before getting out of bed for any reason. Bathing is allowed with advice to have a chair beside the bath to avoid any temptation to stand without the splint. Unless there is a shower seat patients are told not to use a shower. Through the day, patients are encouraged to remove the brace as much as possible while seated to facilitate active ankle exercises. Immediately following fitting of the brace patients attend the physiotherapy department for instruction on active exercise. Where appropriate, the heel raise in the pneumatic walker is reduced after two weeks.

Management Problems

Diagnostic difficulty can arise with a calf muscle tear, as the presenting history is often very similar to that of an Achilles tendon rupture including a description of the sensation of a kick or blow to the back of the ankle. Careful examination will usually resolve the diagnosis as there is no palpable gap in the tendon, and the tenderness is usually located either in the medial or lateral head of gastrocnemius. The tendon itself may be tender, but rarely is it as severe as with a tendon rupture. There is also a different distribution of bruising, although this takes some time to develop and is not evident at the acute presentation (Fig. 3). Such patients are best treated with simple elastic support and crutches. Gradual weight-bearing is allowed as tolerated, and ankle exercises are encouraged with the assistance of a physiotherapist.

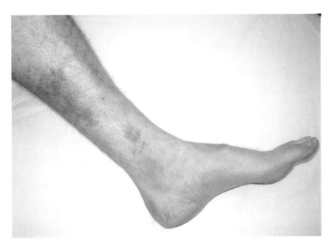

Fig. 3: distribution of bruising in case of calf muscle tear

Incomplete rupture will present with a similar history to that of a complete rupture and a palpable defect. However, plantar flexion power is greater than could be explained by action of the other calf muscles alone. Nevertheless, these patients can be managed using the protocol as for a complete rupture of the tendon. Patients with an incomplete rupture can present late, and this may lead to difficulties with management. In these patients, ultrasonography can help to clarify how much of the tendon remains intact. Any decision to manage surgically is made on clinical grounds rather than relying on diagnostic imaging. The patient's age, level of activity, expectations and general medical status will all have to be taken into account.

Simultaneous bilateral Achilles tendon ruptures can be managed conservatively. A wheelchair is required while both legs are in short leg equinus casts, and, if good family support is not available, hospital admission will be required. Staged removal of the casts and provision of the pneumatic walker one week apart is advised. This is again adopted when the splints are to be removed and free weight bearing commenced.

Patients presenting late are in general not suitable for conservative management. At surgery, the tendon ends are separated by organising haematoma and frequently have become adherent to the adjacent tissues.

Conclusion

This protocol of conservative management can be adopted successfully for routine management of acute Achilles tendon ruptures at all ages and levels of athletic activity. However, the supervising clinician must be sufficiently experienced in this method of management to customise the protocol where appropriate and be able to decide when surgical intervention is required. Furthermore, the supervising clinician should be experienced in such surgery.

Conservative management must not be regarded as an easy management option. To achieve the good results, which can reasonably be expected, close supervision by a senior and experienced clinician is essential. Deviations from the protocol timings may be appropriate in some patients, but require considerable experience.

Whether management is conservative or operative probably the most important aspect of management is the protected active mobilisation of the ankle joints.

References

1] Aldam CH. Repair of calcaneal tendon ruptures. A safe technique. J Bone and Joint Surg 1989;71-B:486-488.

2] Arner O, Lindholm A. Subcutaneous rupture of the Achilles tendon. A study of 92 cases. Acta Chiropractor Scandinavica 1959;239:1-51.

3] Beskin J, Saunders R, Hunter SC, Hughston J. Surgical repair of Achilles tendon ruptures. Am J Sports Med 1987;15:1-8.

4] Bradley JP, Tibone JE. Percutaneous and open surgical repairs of Achilles tendon ruptures. A comparative study. Am J Sports Med 1990; 18:188-195.

5] Cetti R, Henriksen LO, Jacobsen KS. Operative versus nonoperative treatment of the Achilles tendon rupture. A prospective randomized study and review of the literature. Am J Sports Med 1993;21:791-799.

6] Eames MHA, Eames NWA, McCarthy KR, Wallace RGH. An audit of the combined non-operative and orthotic management of ruptured Achilles tendon. Injury 1997;28:289-292.

7] McComis GP, Nawoczenski DA, DeHaven KE. Functional bracing for rupture of the Achilles tendon. Clinical results and analysis of ground-reaction forces and temporal data. J Bone and Joint Surg 1997;79-A:1799-1808.

8] Möller M, Movin T, Granhed K, Lind K, Faxén E, Karlsson J. Acute Rupture of tendo Achillis. A prospective, randomised study of comparison between surgical and non-surgical treatment. J Bone and Joint Surg 2001;83-B:843-848.

9] Nistor L. Surgical and non-surgical treatment of Achilles tendon rupture. A prospective randomised study. J Bone and Joint Surg 1981;63-A:394-398.

10] Stein SR, Leukens CA. Closed treatment of Achilles tendon ruptures. Orthopaedic Clinics of North America 1976;7:241-246.

11] Wallace RGH, Traynor IER, Kernohan WG, Eames MHA. Combined conservative and orthotic management of acute ruptures of the Achilles tendon. J Bone and Joint Surg 2004; 86-A:1198-1202.

Chapter 10.

ULTRASONOGRAPHY-GUIDED MANAGEMENT

H. Thermann

Take Home Message

• *Dynamic ultrasound evaluation enables, by measuring the gapping in plantar-flexion, decision making information about the application of non –operative or operative treatment.*
• *Ultrasound guided treatment in non-operative therapy confirms complete adaptation and therefore "normal" tendon healing in the 4 and 8 weeks follow-up.*
• *Delayed normal tendon healing, tendon stumps separation during healing can be identified during follow-up ultrasound evaluation and appropriate measures (i.e. surgery, prolonged tendon protection) can be carried out.*

Diagnostics

A palpable gap and a positive calf squeeze test are the most important clinical signs of an acute Achilles tendon rupture. The strength of plantar flexion is typically decreased, which results in an inability of single leg heel-raise and impossibility to push off during normal gait, with an externally rotated foot. Some patients are still able to actively plantar flex the foot. This does not indicate an intact Achilles tendon, as the long toe flexors, such as the flexor digitorum longus and flexor hallucis longus, are still working.

Although most Achilles tendon ruptures can be diagnosed clinically, evaluation by ultrasonography and MRI may be used to guide management. The ultrasonographic appearance of an acute Achilles tendon rupture is very variable. The most common signs are interruption of continuity, with well defined tendon stumps. Hypoechogenic accumulation of fluid at the rupture site and loss of the typical parallel hyperechogenicity pattern are identified regularly by experienced examiners. As some ruptures do not show a visible gap between the proximal and distal stumps from organisation of the haematoma, dynamic examination in dorsiflexion and plantar flexion is recommended. Even though no gap is identified, the loss of the well ordered appearance of the collagen network reveals a rupture. Tendinopathic changes, with increased antero-posterior diameter and loss of the intratendinous structure, but maintenance of tendon continuity, have to be identified.

At times, imaging reports a partial rupture. In these instances, clinical examination revealing loss of function of the Achilles/Soleus/Gastrocnemius complex with inability of single–leg toe raise will guide the diagnosis.

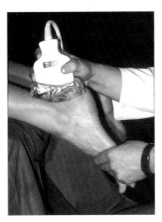 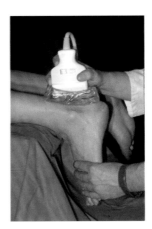

Fig. 1: Sonographic examination in 20° plantarflexion and neutral position

Management

Non-surgical management

Simple immobilisation in a cast is not justified, given the documented deleterious effects of of muscle hypotrophy and loss of coordination, proprioception and joint stiffness. We use ultrasound or MRI as a basis for management strategy.

1. If the there is ultrasonographic or MRI evidence of juxtaposition of the tendon stumps with the foot at 20° of plantar flexion, we undertake conservative management. If ultrasonography or MRI shows gapping between the tendon stumps, we prefer surgical management, or, if patients still require conservative management, we inform them that this may lead to higher risk of rerupture, or result in a weak Gastroc/Soleus complex.

2. As non-operative management cannot mechanically stabilise the tendon stumps, if patients are mobile even well juxtaposed tendon stumps may separate and a secondary gap develops. Therefore, we recommend a further ultrasonography exam after 4 weeks to ascertain whether the tendon is healing normally. Clinically, at that stage there should be full palpable continuity of the tendon. Asking the patient to performing plantar flexion against minimal resistance should produce slight tensioning of the gastrocnemii. At ultrasonography, the restored continuity of the tendon should be evident as a dishomogeneous structure with echogenic and hypogenic areas, with an antero-posterior diameter of 6 to 10 mm.

3. At 8 weeks, the protecting orthosis or therapy walker or boots is discarded. We recommend a final ultrasonography check at this stage. Usually, at this stage the antero-posterior diameter of the tendon is 10 to 14 mm. Ultrasonography shows greater structural alignment of the collagen fibres. Clinically a broad, stable tendon is palpable, the calf squeeze test is negative, and in plantarflexion the patient can exert moderate power against resistance. If deficient tendon healing has occurred, with an hourglass appearance at the rupture side, further imaging is required.

4. If ultrasonography at 4 weeks shows gapping of the stumps, the tendon will heal with elongation. In these instances, we perform a percutaneous suture of the Achilles tendon. The treatment in the orthosis/ boot is then continued for another 8 weeks, with ultrasonographical checks at 4 and 8 weeks.

5. Gapping after 8 weeks of conservative management implies delayed healing, and requires further protection for another 2 to 4 weeks. In a prospective ultrasonography study, we have found an increase of the tendon callus following functional treatment from the 6th to the 12th week, with a peak at 10 weeks. In patients with systemic co-morbidities (i.e., spontaneous rupture after heart or kidney transplantation), we have seen regeneration of the tendon at 6 months during which time the patients have used a therapy boot.

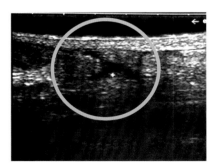 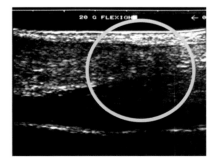

Fig. 2: Gapping in 0° and complete tendon adaptation at 20° plantarflexion

Rehabilitation

The appropriate orthosis with heel rise plays major role in rehabilitation and in regaining functional ability. The orthosis prevents stress at the rupture site while allowing axial loading, which promotes tendon healing.

The orthosis prevents dorsiflexion; the lateral shaft stabilizer reduces torsional stresses, and the heel pads allow gradual adjustment from 20° from plantar flexion to the neutral position. With the fitted orthosis, patients are allowed to weight bear fully, and to continue their activities of daily living according to pain and swelling.

Patients wear the orthosis for 6 weeks, day and night (or alternatively a night splint to protect the tendon), and for a further 2 weeks only during the day. After three weeks with the fitted orthosis, patients are allowed to exercise on a stationary bike against little resistance. In athletes, after 4 weeks increased physiotherapy is allowed, with progressive strengthening exercises (isometric exercises, isokinetic bicycle), proprioceptive neuromuscular facilitation (PNF), and coordination exercises in the orthosis. In addition, ultrasound application (1 MHz) and cryotherapy can be performed to enhance tendon healing.

After 8 weeks, an ultrasonographic check evaluates tendon healing. If this is adequate, the orthosis is discarded. A small heel lift in a normal shoe is recommended for a further 6 to 8 weeks. Jogging is allowed after 3 month if coordination and muscle strength are appropriate.

At that stage, the antero-posterior diameter of the tendon is 16-20 mm, about 2.5-3 times the normal size of the Achilles tendon. Jogging and low impact activities are allowed if the antero-posterior diameter of the tendon is 12-14 mm after 4 to 5 month. It normally takes about one year to regaining pre-injury status.

Evidence based medicine

There are several meta-analyses on Achilles tendon rupture[2,6,11,13,15]. These do not consider the juxtaposition of the tendon stumps as a criterion to guide management. Kotnis and co-workers[12] performed a retrospective study with the same dynamic ultrasound selection for non-operative versus open surgery. The results were similar, which shows the effectiveness of ultrasound guidance in Achilles tendon ruptures.

References

1] Arner O, Lindholm A. Subcutaneous rupture of the Achilles tendon; a study of 92 cases. Acta Chir Scand Suppl 1959;116:1-51.
2] Bhandari M, Guyatt GH, Siddiqui F, et al. Treatment of acute Achilles tendon ruptures: a systematic overview and meta-analysis. Clin Orthop Relat Res 2002:190-200.
3] Buchgraber A, Paessler HH. Percutaneous repair of Ahilles tendon rupture. Immobilization versus functional postoperative treatment. Clin Orthop 1997;341:113-122.
4] Cetti R, Christensen SE, Ejsted R, Jensen NM, Jorgensen U. Operative versus nonoperative treatment of Achilles tendon rupture. A prospective randomized study and review of the literature. Am J Sports Med 1993;21:791-799.

5] Christensen J. Rupture Achilles tendon. Acta Chir Scand 1953;106.

6] Dobson MH, Nguyen C. Treatment of acute Achilles tendon ruptures. A meta-analysis of randomized, controlled trials. J Bone Joint Surg Am 2005;87:1160.

7] Inglis AE, Scuco TP. Surgical repair of ruptures of the tendo Achillis. Clin Orthop 1981;156:160-169.

8] Jacobs D, Martens M, Van Audekercke R, Mulier JC, Mulier F. Comparison of conservative and operative treatment of Achilles tendon rupture. Am J Sports Med 1978;6:107-111.

9] Jozsa L, Kvist M, Balint BJ, et al. The role of recreational sport activity in Achilles tendon rupture. A clinical, pathoanatomical, and sociological study of 292 cases. Am J Sports Med 1989;17:338-343.

10] Kannus P, Jozsa L. Histopathological changes preceding spontaneous rupture of a tendon. A controlled study of 891 patients. J Bone Joint Surg Am 1991;73:1507-1525.

11] Khan RJ, Fick D, Keogh A, Crawford J, Brammar T, Parker M. Treatment of acute achilles tendon ruptures. A meta-analysis of randomized, controlled trials. J Bone Joint Surg Am 2005;87:2202-2210.

12] Kotnis R, David S, Handley,R, Willett K, Ostlere S. Dynamic ultrasound as a selection tool for reducing Achilles tendon ruptures. AJSM 2006;34;1395-1400.

13] Lo IK, Kirkley A, Nonweiler B, Kumbhare DA. Operative versus nonoperative treatment of acute Achilles tendon ruptures: a quantitative review. Clin J Sport Med 1997;7:207-211.

14] McComis GP, Nawoczenski DA, DeHaven KE. Functional bracing for rupture of the Achilles tendon. Clinical results and analysis of ground-reaction forces and temporal data. J Bone Joint Surg Am 1997;79:1799-1808.

15] McCormack RG. Treatment of acute Achilles tendon ruptures: a systematic overview and metaanalysis. Clin J Sport Med 2003;13:194.

16] Nistor L. Surgical and non-surgical treatment of Achilles Tendon rupture. A prospective randomized study. J Bone Joint Surg Am 1981;63:394-399.

17] Riede D. [Comments on "Therapy and late results of subcutaneous Achilles tendon rupture". Beitr Orthop Traumatol 1972;19:328-331.

18] Schonbauer HR. Diseases of the Achilles tendon. Wien Klin Wochenschr Suppl 1986;168:1-47.

19] Thermann H, Zwipp H, Tscherne H. Functional treatment concept of acute rupture of the Achilles tendon. 2 years results of a prospective randomized study. Unfallchirurg 1995:98:21-32.

20] Thermann H. Rupture of the Achilles tendon--conservative functional treatment. Z Orthop Ihre Grenzgeb 1998;136:20-22.

21] Thermann H. Treatment of Achilles tendon rupture. Unfallchirurg 1998;101:299-314.

22] Thermann H. Treatment of Achilles tendon ruptures. Foot and Ankle Clinics 1999;4:773-787.

*"Start by doing what's necessary,
then what's possible and suddenly
you are doing the impossible."*

(St. Francis of Assisi)

Chapter 11.

CHRONIC RUPTURES

Murali K. Sayana, Masato Takao, Nicola Maffulli

Take Home Message

• *Conservative management is not recommended for chronic Achilles tendon ruptures.*
• *The Achilles tendon should be reconstructed to a functional length using turn-down slip or slips, peroneus brevis tendon, flexor hallucis longus tendon, or a free graft of one of the hamstring tendons or a free gastrocnemius flap.*
• *Augmentation with plantaris tendon and/or interposed scar tissue may be beneficial for a firm connection between the distal and proximal stumps, which allows an accelerated rehabilitation after surgery and maturity of the reconstructed tendon.*

Introduction

Chronic Achilles tendon ruptures are relatively uncommon, and are defined as a rupture of the Achilles tendon with an interval between rupture and treatment of at least 4 to 6 weeks. In such patients, the triceps surae is shortened, and the gap between the proximal and distal stumps of the Achilles tendon can be filled up with fibrous tissue. Thus, the strength of plantar flexion of the ankle is affected. Active plantar flexion at the ankle occurs thanks to the action of secondary plantar flexors of the ankle joint. Therefore, the aim of management of chronic Achilles tendon ruptures is to reconstruct the Achilles tendon to a functional length and achieve normal plantar flexion strength. Incidence of re-rupture after initial surgical management has reported to be 1.7% to 5.4% and after conservative management is 12.7% to 20.8% [11]. Reruptures can be considered as a chronic ruptures, as debridement to healthy margins may leave a considerable gap between the stumps.

Diagnosis

1. Clinical examination

Clinical examination alone is sufficient for a clinician to diagnose an acute Achilles tendon rupture. That may not be the case in a chronic rupture, as pain and swelling have often subsided, with the gap between the tendon ends filled in with fibrous tissue[15,16]. The calf muscles can be wasted. The long toe flexors may try and compensate for the lack of function of the gastrocnemius/soleus complex, producing clawing of the toes and an apparently high medial arch of the foot[18]. Although some active plantarflexion is produced by the action of the long flexors of the foot, and by the concerted action of tibialis posterior and the peronei, a single leg tip toe raise on the involved leg is impossible. Patients have increased dorsiflexion at the ankle to due absence of intact triceps surae mechanism. Plantar flexion strength is always reduced. Calf squeeze tests (Simmond's and Matle's) may be of dubious interpretation, and it is always important to compare with the healthy leg. Imaging may have to be used to confirm the diagnosis, but may sometimes be difficult to interpret.

2. Imaging

Lateral radiographs of the ankle may demonstrate distortion of the Kager triangle and/or calcification of the distal stump of the Achilles tendon (Figure 1). Ultrasonography of a neglected rupture will reveal an acoustic vacuum with thick irregular edges[14,16]. Magnetic resonance imaging will reveal generalised high signal intensity on T2 weighted images. On T1 weighted images, the rupture will appear as a disruption of the signal within the tendon substance[10] (Figure 2).

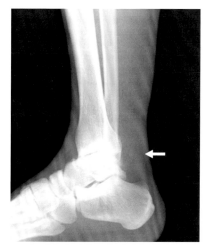

Figure 1: Lateral radiograph of the ankle in a case of chronic Achilles tendon rupture
An arrow shows a distortion of Kager's triangle.

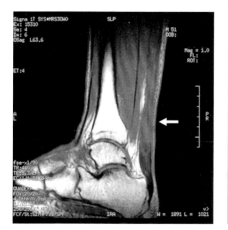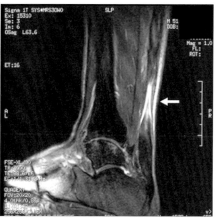

Figure 2: MR imaging in a case of chronic Achilles tendon rupture
On T1 weighted images (left), the rupture appears as a disruption of the signal within the tendon substance (arrow). On T2 weighted images (right), it reveals high signal intensity (arrow).

Classification

Two classification systems have been proposed[12,20]. Both use the length of the tendon defect as the basis for management (Table 1).

A. Myerson's classification system[20]
1. Defects of 1 to 2 cm are managed with end-to-end repair and posterior compartment fasciotomy.
2. Defects between 2 and 5 cm are repaired using V-Y lengthening +/- tendon transfer.
3. Defects greater than 5 cm are repaired using tendon transfer alone or in combination with V-Y advancement.
B. Kuwada's classification system[12]
Type I: Partial ruptures are managed with plaster cast immobilisation.
Type II: Complete ruptures with defects up to 3 cm are managed with end-to-end repair.
Type III: Complete ruptures with 3-6 cm defects after debridement of tendon ends to healthy tissue are managed with tendon graft/flap +/- augmentation with synthetic graft.
Type IV: Complete ruptures with defect over 6 cm after debridement of tendon ends to healthy tissue are managed with gastrocnemius recession, a free tendon graft and/or synthetic tendon graft.

Table 1: Classification systems of chronic Achilles tendon ruptures

Pathophysiology

The tendon sheath often becomes thickened and adherent to the retracted tendon ends, without much functional repair tissue between the torn ends[14,20]. The proximal tendon stump is often conical and the distal stump often looks bulbous. The plantaris tendon may be hypertrophied if present. Retraction of the proximal stump results in shortening of the gastrocnemius/soleus complex, which thereby reduces the biomechanical efficiency and the contractile force which the muscle can develop.

Management

Management of chronic Achilles tendon ruptures is more challenging than that of acute ruptures.

1. Conservative management

Conservative management, although a consideration is not recommended. In rabbits[23], a well organised connective tissue was seen at 56 days after their calcaneal tendons resection. By 240 days, however, it still did not display the fascicular arrangement of a tendon. This new tissue was not as strong as intact tendon, and it elongated with time[3,20]. Christensen and co-workers[5] showed that satisfactory results were obtained in 10 of 18 (56%) of non-operated patients. In addition, improvement in all non-operated patients occurred slowly, sometimes over several years. This compared poorly with the patients managed surgically. A brace or ankle/foot orthosis was also reported as beneficial.

2. Surgical management

Percutaneous repair is usually not possible, and is not considered a valid option. An open procedure must be performed[12]. Even the open procedure is different from acute rupture, as the tendon ends would have retracted, and typically require debridement of interposed scar tissue.
The blood supply to this area is poor, and the tendon ends have to be freshened to allow for the repair healing. However, due to the increased gap, primary repair may be difficult. Direct end-to-end repair of the tendon ends can only be possible by exceeding the ankle's physiological equinus. However, this is not a problem in the long term, and if the repair is sound, then early mobilisation can be implemented, and return to a normal range on motion, including physiological dorsiflexion, can usually be obtained by three to five months from the procedure.
Numerous techniques to reconstruct the chronic Achilles tendon rupture have been reported. To re-establish tendon continuity, surgeons may consider using: (1) the residual Achilles tendon, (2) adjacent flexor tendons, and (3) free grafts.

2.1 Residual Achilles tendon

A turn-down procedure utilizes a central slip (Figure 3)[3], or medial and lateral flaps (Figure 4)[13], of the proximal Achilles tendon to bridge the gap. It is harvested through a posterior longitudinal incision and dissected as approximately 10-15 mm by 15 to 18 cm strip of tendon on a distal pedicle. The strip is threaded through the trimmed ends of the ruptured tendon and sutured to them with the foot in plantarflexion. Alternatively, a proximal-to-distal V-Y advancement of the gastrocnemius tendon has also been described[1].

Some members of the Achilles Tendon Study Group routinely use a direct repair by means of the triple bundle technique in chronic Achilles tendon tears of up to one year duration.

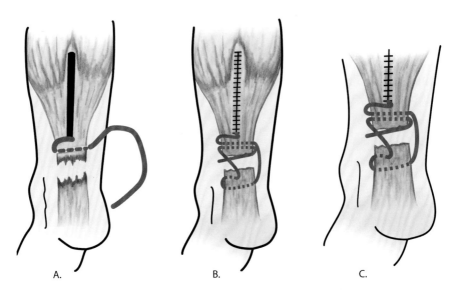

A.   B.   C.

Figure 3: A turndown procedure utilizing a central slip described by Bosworth[3]

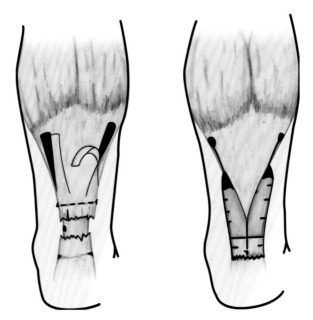

Figure 4: A turndown procedure utilizing the medial and lateral slips described by Lindholm[13]

2.2 Adjacent tendons

The tendon of flexor hallucis longus (FHL) has been used because it is a long tendon that will allow bridging of large Achilles tendon defects[25]. It is weaved through the ruptured Achilles tendon ends. The distal stump of the FHL tendon is tenodesed to the tendon of flexor digitorum longus (FDL) of the second toe. Each patient developed a "small but functionally insignificant loss in range of motion in the involved ankle and great toe". This may be important in athletic individuals, in whom the loss of push-off from the hallux may cause difficulty when sprinting. Peroneus brevis tendon transfer for rupture of the Achilles tendon was popularised by Perez-Teuffer (Figure 5)[22]. In the original technique, the harvested peroneus brevis tendon was passed through a transosseous drill hole in the calcaneus. McClelland and Maffulli[19] approached the Achilles tendon medially, and deliver the peroneus brevis tendon through the postero-medial wound. Although all these patients were satisfied with the procedure, they had greater loss of isokinetic strength variables at high speeds and greater loss of calf circumference when compared with patients who underwent open repair of fresh Achilles tendon rupture.

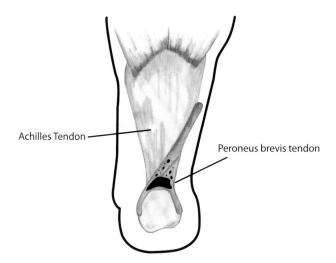

Achilles Tendon

Peroneus brevis tendon

Figure 5: Peroneus brevis transfer described by Perez-Teuffer[22]

2.3 Free Grafts

Fascia lata grafts, plantaris, hamstring tendons, free gastrocnemius aponeurosis and synthetic materials have also been used in the management of neglected or chronic ruptures of the Achilles tendon. The gracilis tendon can also be used as a free graft to bridge the gap[17], if the gap produced after debriding the scar tissue is greater than 6 cm despite maximal plantar flexion of the ankle and traction on the Achilles tendon stumps.

2.4 Augmentation with interposed scar tissue

Simultaneous augmentation may be beneficial for the maturity of the recon-structed tendons. The tendon of plantaris, if present, can be harvested to aug-ment the repair if there is a large gap. Yasuda and co-workers[26] noted that the thick fibrous scar tissue found between the two ruptured ends of Achilles tendon was strong enough to resist significant tensile forces. They resected the middle third of the interposed scar tissue, and sutured the two free ends of Achilles ten-don. Histological examination of the resected tissue showed dense collagen fi-bres with blood vessels and no degenerative changes.

Post-operative management

No studies have been published that focussed specifically on post-operative management following surgery for chronic Achilles tendon ruptures. If satis-factory approximation/adequate repair of the distal and proximal stumps is achieved intra-operatively, accelerated rehabilitation, presently recommended in acute tears, is beneficial[24].

Complications

Wound infection, wound haematoma and breakdown, hypersensitivity of the surgical wounds, sural nerve sensory deficit, re-rupture, DVT are all risks with open repair or reconstruction chronic rupture of the Achilles tendon.
If a longitudinal incision is used in open repair of the Achilles tendon, it passes through poorly vascularised skin[7], with the potential of poorly healing wounds. This risk can be reduced by careful handling of tissues and by maintaining thick skin flaps throughout the procedure. Even small defects take a long time to heal. Wounds that break down need coverage, as tendons left exposed undergo desic-cation and secondary adhesions. Complications have to be recognised early, and should receive expedient appropriate management. The medial longitudinal in-cision helps avoid damage to the sural nerve.
Although re-ruptures are rare[22], patients should be advised that the risk is present and should be cautioned about careful re-mobilisation after discarding the cast.

Further suggestions

Nellas and co-workers[21] used two strips of freeze dried Achilles tendon allograft to reconstruct a 4.5 cm tendon defect. That patient had a good functional re-sult, although peak torques were lower compared with the uninjured side. More recently, Haraguchi and co-workers[8] performed Achilles tendon allografts for chronic Achilles tendon ruptures. No formal results have been published, but nei-ther allograft rejection nor transmission of any disease to the host has occurred. Tissue engineering may prove useful for managing tendon ruptures. A 1 cm long gap injury model in rabbit Achilles tendon was used to compare suture alone with a cell-collagen gel composite that was contracted onto a pre-tensioned suture[9]. Evaluation at 4, 8, and 12 weeks following surgery revealed that structural and material properties of the cell-treated implants typically were approximately twice the value of controls. Cell-treated repairs were larger in cross-section and better organized histologically than repairs that were done with suture alone. Window defects in rabbit patellar tendons were treated with autologous mesenchymal stem cells (MSCs) that were seeded onto a collagen implant, whereas unseeded collagen implants were placed into the control limb[4]. At 4 weeks, the MSC repairs had greater maximum stress (26%) and strain energy density (33%) than matched control. Such an approach could be used in patients with chronic Achilles rupture.

Tissue engineering is an emerging field, and many difficulties need to be overcome before this becomes a realistic option in the management of tendon disorders. It is important to determine whether effective vascularisation and innervations of implanted tissue-engineered constructs takes place. Vascularisation is important for the viability of the construct. Innervation is required for proprioception and to maintain reflexes that are mediated by Golgi tendon organs to protect tendons from excessive forces[2].

References

1] Abraham E, Pankovich AM. Neglected rupture of the Achilles tendon. Treatment by V-Y tendinous flap. J Bone Joint Surg Am 1975;57-A:253-255.

2] Baechle, T.R. and Earle, R.W. Essentials of strength training and conditioning. 2nd edition. Champaign, IL: National Strength and Conditioning Association, 2000.

3] Bosworth DM. Repair of defects in the Tendo Achillis. J Bone Joint Surg Am 1956;38-A;111-114.

4] Cao Y, Liu Y, Liu W, Shan, Q, Buonocore S D, Cui L. Bridging tendon defects using autologous tenocyte engineered tendon in a hen model. Plast Reconstr Surg 2002;110:1280-9.

5] Christensen I. Rupture of the Achilles tendon; analysis of 57 cases. Acta Chir Scand 1953;106:50-60.

6] Gabel S, Manoli A. Neglected rupture of the Achilles tendon. Foot Ankle Int, 1994;15:512-517.

7] Haertsch PA. The blood supply of the skin of the leg: a post-mortem investigation. Br J Plast Surg 1981;34:470-477.

8] Haraguchi N, Bluman EM, Myerson MS. Reconstruction of chronic Achilles tendon disorders with Achilles tendon allograft. Techniques in Foot & Ankle Surgery, 2005;4:154-159.

9] He Q, Li Q, Chen B, Wang Z. Repair of flexor tendon defects of rabbit with tissue engineering method. Chin J Traumatol 2002;5:200-208.

10] Kabbani YM, Mayer DP. Magnetic resonance imaging of tendon pathology about the foot and ankle. Part I. Achilles tendon. J Am Podiatr Med Ass 1993;83:418-420.

11] Khan RJ, Fick D, Keogh A, Crawford J, Brammar T, Parker M. Treatment of acute achilles tendon ruptures. A meta-analysis of randomized, controlled trials. J Bone Joint Surg Am 2005;87:2202-2210.

12] Kuwada GT. Classification of tendo Achillis rupture with consideration of surgical repair techniques. J Foot Surg, 1990;29:361-365.

13] Lindholm A. A new method of operation in subcutaneous rupture of the Achilles tendon. Acta Chir Scandinavica, 1959; 117:261-270.

14] Maffulli N, Dymond NP, Capasso G. Ultrasonographic findings in subcutaneous rupture of Achilles tendon. J Sports Med Phys Fitness 1989;29:365-368.

15] Maffulli N. The clinical diagnosis of subcutaneous tear of the Achilles tendon. A prospective study in 174 patients. Am J Sports Med 1998;26:266-270.

16] Maffulli N. Rupture of the Achilles tendon. J Bone Joint Surg Am 1999; 81-A:1019-1036.

17] Maffulli N, Leadbetter WB. Free Gracilis Tendon Graft in Neglected Tears of the Achilles Tendon.

Clin J Sport Med 2005;15:56-61.

18] Mann RA, Holmes GB, Seale KS et al. Chronic rupture of the Achilles tendon: a new technique of repair. J Bone Joint Surg Am 1991;73-A:214-219.

19] McClelland D, Maffulli N. Neglected rupture of the Achilles tendon: reconstruction with peroneus brevis tendon transfer. Surgeon 2004;2:209-213.

20] Myerson MS. Achilles tendon ruptures. Instr Course Lect, 1999;48:219-230.

21] Nellas ZJ, Loder BG, Wertheimer SJ. Reconstruction of an Achilles tendon defect utilizing an Achilles tendon allograft. J Foot Ankle Surg 1996;35:144-148.

22] Perez-Teuffer A. Traumatic rupture of the Achilles tendon. Reconstruction by transplant and graft using the lateral peroneus brevis. Orthop Clin North Am 1974;5:89-93.

23] Postacchini F, Accinni L, Natali PG, Ippolito E, DeMartino C. Regeneration of rabbit calcaneal tendon: a morphological and immunochemical study. Cell Tissue Res 1978;195:81-97.

24] Takao M, Ochi M, Naito K, Uchio Y, Matsusaki M, Oae K. Repair of neglected Achilles tendon rupture using gastrocnemius fascial flaps. Arch Orthop Trauma Surg 2003;123:471-474.

25] Wapner KL, Pavlock GS, Hecht PJ, et al. Repair of chronic Achilles tendon rupture with Flexor hallucis longus tendon transfer. Foot Ankle 1993;14:443-449.

26] Yasuda T, Kinoshita M, Okuda R. Reconstruction of chronic Achilles tendon rupture with the use of interposed tissue between the stumps. Am J Sports Med 2007;35:582-588.

"The Achilles tendon, if bruised or cut, causes the most acute fevers, induces choking, deranges the mind, and at length brings death."

(Hippocrates)

Chapter 12.

STRENGTH, ELONGATION AND HEEL RAISE

Karsten Knobloch

Take Home Message

• *Strength is significantly deteriorated following Achilles tendon rupture with the need for a thorough long-term strength training.*
• *Early functional treatment following surgical repair of the Achilles tendon is associated with beneficial functional outcomes.*
• *Proprioceptive training following Achilles tendon repair appears to be attractive, but has to be studied in further prospective randomized trials.*

Introduction

The Achilles tendon is the largest tendon in the body. Total resection of the Achilles tendon, such as following complicated Achilles tendon infection with radical debridement, results in a plantar flexion force of 45% on the resected side in comparison to the healthy side[1]. It has been reported that surgery for Achilles tendinopathy leads to persisting side-to-side differences in calf muscle strength[12]. As such, concentric plantar flexion peak torque at 90°/sec and 225°/sec and eccentric plantar flexion peak torque at 90°/sec were still significantly lower (7.2%, 8.6% and 8.8% respectively) on the injured side compared to the non-injured side five years after surgery. However, the percentage side-to-side difference was relatively low, and might not have any clinical relevance.

Strength

Currently there is no consensus regarding the best method to determine strength. Strength testing has been performed using isokinetic dynamometry, which has been reported with reliability slightly greater on the healthy side (0.74-0.92 ICC) in comparison with the injured side (0.74-0.89 ICC) among 22 subjects 6 months following Achilles tendon rupture[2]. Kin-com Dynamometer was used to measure the torque of the plantar flexors. Twelve subjects had been managed operatively and 10 non-operatively. Subjects were placed in the prone position with the knee extended. Measurements of peak torque, average torque, and total work were made for both concentric and eccentric plantar flexion movements at 60°/sec.

Isokinetic strength and endurance are similar following open surgery and percutaneous repair for acute ruptures of the Achilles tendon[5]. An isokinetic Biodex dynamometer (Biodex Medical System, Shirley, NY) was used to measure ankle joint angle, and in plantarflexion to calculate the torque at the ankle joint (Newton/meter), as well as the average work (Joules) for both maximal power and endurance. Biodex dynamometer evaluations at 90°/sec demonstrated a significant difference of maximal voluntary plantar flexor torque, endurance performance and range of motion at the ankle joint between the involved and uninvolved sides irrespective of the selected treatment. Yet, no statistically significant differences were shown in the above variables between the subjects who received either percutaneous or open surgery.

Disproportionate weakness in end-range plantar flexion, decreased passive stiffness in dorsiflexion, and inability to perform a decline heel-rise are evident after Achilles tendon repair[11]. Significant plantar flexion weakness was evident on the involved side at 10° and 20° of plantar flexion (20% and 34% deficits, respectively; p<.001), with no torque deficits evident at other angles (6% at neutral, 3% at 10° of dorsiflexion, 0% at 20° of dorsiflexion). Impairments will have functional implications for activities (e.g., descending stairs and landing from a jump). Four-strand core suture repairs of Achilles tendon were performed on 1 female patient and 19 male patients. Postoperatively, patients were non-weight bearing with the ankle immobilized for 4 weeks. Plantar flexion torque, dorsiflexion range of motion, passive joint stiffness, toe walking, and standing single-legged heel rise (on an incline, decline, and level surface) were assessed at a mean 1.8 years after surgery (range: 6 months-9 years). Weakness in end-range plantar flexion may be an unrecognized problem after Achilles tendon repair.

As far as rehabilitation following Achilles tendon ruptures is concerned a meta-analysis stated that early functional treatment protocols, when compared with postoperative immobilization, led to superior subjective functional outcome and no difference in rerupture rate[13]. However, these conclusions were based on six trials with small sample sizes, and larger randomized trials are required to confirm these results.

Based on a randomized controlled trial, the isokinetic calf muscle strength results are better in an early motion group following Achilles tendon rupture vs. an immobilisation group, whereas the other outcomes in these two groups of patients were similar[7]. Fifty patients with an acute Achilles tendon rupture were randomized postoperatively to receive either early movement of the ankle between neutral and plantar flexion in a brace for 6 weeks, or Achilles tendon immobilization in tension using a below-knee cast with the ankle in a neutral position for 6 weeks. Full weight bearing was allowed after 3 weeks in both groups. The patients were assessed clinically at 1, 3, 6, 12, and 24 weeks, and the last control visit took place at a mean of 60 weeks postoperatively. The isokinetic calf muscle strength scores were excellent in 56%, good in 32%, fair in 8%, and poor in 4% of the patients in the early motion group at the last follow-up examination. The scores in the cast group were excellent in 29%, good in 50%, and fair in 21% of the patients.

Functional assessment of the outcome of reconstructed Achilles tendons should involve gait analysis. Recently, improvement in gait pattern has been reported to be slower than recovery of plantar flexor mechanical properties in 49 young adults (27 men and 22 women) who underwent surgical repair of a complete Achilles tendon rupture[4]. At 24 months, a deficit in calf-muscle eccentric strength was still present, determining adaptive changes in gait strategy, involving ankle motion and coordinated muscular activity. Persisting mechanical impairment 24 months after surgery resulting in gait adaptations may be detrimental to the healing structures by increasing stress on the Achilles tendon. Accordingly, restoration of calf-muscle eccentric strength and coordinated antagonist muscle activity should be key points in postoperative rehabilitation following surgical repair of Achilles tendon rupture. A proprioceptive training intervention, besides eccentric training, may proof beneficial in this regard. However, currently randomized-controlled trials on this issue are pending, but are worthwhile to consider.

Elongation

As far as Achilles tendon elongation is considered, there is no clear definition and no validated outcome measure for tendon elongation at all. Typically, tendon elongation is evaluated by inspection followed by range of motion of the ankle. Increased dorsiflexion following an Achilles tendon tear irrespective of the mode of treatment (functional or surgical) might be evidenced in patients with Achilles tendon elongation in contrast to what found on the contralateral uninjured side. Furthermore, one could determine tendon elongation using the difference in the height of the gastrocnemius muscle belly. However, none of these methods have been validated.

Disproportionate weakness in end-range plantar flexion, decreased passive stiffness in dorsiflexion, and inability to perform a decline heel rise are evident after Achilles tendon repair[11]. Significant plantarflexion weakness was evident on the involved side at 10° and 20° of plantar flexion (20% and 34% deficits, respectively; p <.001), with no torque deficits evident at other angles (6% at neutral, 3% at 10° of dorsiflexion, 0% at 20° of dorsiflexion). Impairments will have functional implications for activities (e.g. descending stairs and landing from a jump). Therefore, tendon training as achieved by an eccentric training might proof beneficial among patients suffering Achilles tendon ruptures in the rehabilitation period. However, trials are pending especially regarding the best point of time to start with the eccentric training in the rehabilitation period.

Heel raise

Given that the use of a heel raise during rehabilitation following Achilles tendon repair relieves strain on the Achilles tendon, one has to question the extent and the duration of heel rise in a given rehabilitation protocol. Early functional rehabilitation, as performed in hand surgery for extensor and flexor tendon injuries, has been proposed following Achilles tendon surgery with favourable outcome. Heel rise is a potential strain relieving measure might be an appropriate option at a given time with a given extent. However, to date no randomized-controlled trials are available regarding various regimens of heel-rise protocols to recommend a detailed protocol. Often, heel-rise is part of modern orthoses [8]. The rehabilitation protocol at the Hannover Medical School, Germany involves heel rise of 3 cm for up to 8 weeks with 1 cm heel rise from week 9-12 depending on ultrasonographic appearance of tendon healing and compliance of the patient. We use the appearance of the Achilles tendon at dynamic ultrasonographic examination at 25° of plantar flexion of the ankle has to be stressed[9]. However, currently there is no level of evidence in this respect.

Given the fact that there seems to be a continuum from the healthy Achilles tendon over tendinopathy to Achilles tendon rupture further, currently undetermined factors might contribute to the success of a given treatment option after Achilles tendon rupture. As such, gender might play a role in this regard since Achilles tendon microcirculation is different among symptomatic females versus male suffering Achilles tendinopathy[10]. Furthermore, hormone replacement therapy has been associated with Achilles tendinopathy[3,6]. The outcome after repair of the ruptured Achilles tendon might therefore at least been influenced by gender. Further studies might address the effects of a given rehabilitation protocol in this respect.

References

1] Boorboor P, Lahoda LU, Spies M, Kuether G, Waehling K, Vogt PM. Resection of infected Achilles tendon. Results after soft tissue coverage without tendon reconstruction. Chirurg 2006;77:1144-1151.

2] Chester R, Costa ML, Shepstone L, Donell ST. Reliability of isokinetic dynamometry in assessing plantarflexion torque following Achilles tendon rupture. Foot Ankle Int 2003;24:909-915.

3] Cook JL, Bass SL, Black JE. Hormone therapy is associated with smaller Achilles tendon diameter in active post-menopausal women. Scand J Med Sci Sports 2007;17:128-132.

4] Don R, Ranavolo A, Cacchio A, Serrao M, Costabile F, Iachelli M, Camerota F, Frascarelli M, Santilli V. Relationship between recovery of calf-muscle biomechanical properties and gait pattern following surgery for achilles tendon rupture. Clin Biomech (Bristol, Avon) 2007;22:211-220.

5] Goren D, Ayalon M, Nyska M. Isokinetic strength and endurance after percutaneous and open surgical repair of Achilles tendon ruptures. Foot Ankle Int 2005;26:286-290.

6] Holmes GB, Lin J. Etiologic factors associated with symptomatic Achilles tendinopathy. Foot Ankle Int 2006;27:952-959.

7] Kangas J, Pajala A, Siira P, Hämäläinen M, Leppilahti J. Early functional treatment versus early immobilization in tension of the musculotendinous unit after Achilles rupture repair: a prospective, randomized, clinical study. J Trauma 2003;54:1171-1181.

8] Knobloch K, Thermann H, Hüfner T. Achilles tendon rupture – early functional and surgical options with special emphasis on rehabilitation issues. Sportverletz Sportschaden 2007;21:34-40.

9] Knobloch K, Thermann H, Hüfner T. Dynamic ultrasound as a selection tool for reducing Achilles tendon reruptures. Am J Sports Med 2007;35:150.

10] Knobloch K, Schreibmueller L, Meller R, Busch KH, Spies M, Vogt PM. Superior Achilles tendon microcirculation in tendinopathy among symptomatic females versus male patients. Am J Sports Med 2007 [Epub ahead of print].

11] Mullaney MJ, McHugh MP, Tyler TF, Nicholas SJ, Lee SJ. Weakness in end-range plantar flexion after Achilles tendon repair. Am J Sports Med 2006 Jul;34:1120-1125.

12] Ohberg L, Lorentzon R, Alfredson H. Good clinical results but persisting side-to-side differences in calf muscle strength after surgical treatment of chronic Achilles tendinosis: a 5-year follow-up. Scand J Med Sci Sports 2001;11:207-212.

13] Suchak AA, Spooner C, Reid DC, Jomha NM. Postoperative rehabilitation protocols for Achilles tendon ruptures: a meta-analysis. Clin Orthop Relat Res 2006;445:216-221.

CHAPTER 13.

THE ROLE OF WEIGHT-BEARING

Murali K. Sayana, Nicola Maffulli

Take Home Message

• *Traditional protocols recommend sequential change of non-weight-bearing casts at 2, 4, 6 weeks after surgery to move the ankle from equinus to the neutral position.*
• *Early weight-bearing after acute Achilles tendon repair is recommended as it improves patient satisfaction with reduction in minor complications and no increase in rerupture or infection rates.*

Introduction

Prolonged Immobilization following musculo-skeletal injury may result in detrimental effects. Lower tensile strength and strain at failure were demonstrated in collagen fascicles from stress shielded rabbit patellar tendons compared with control samples[23]. Immobilization not only reduces the water and proteoglycan content of tendons, but also increases the number of reducible collagen cross-links[1,2].

Early resumption of activity promotes restoration of function, and motion therapy strategies aim to facilitate healing, reduce adhesion formation and increase range of motion[7,8]. Early mobilization following tendon repair is beneficial, and several postoperative mobilization protocols are advocated[9,11,12]. Repetitive motion results in increased DNA content and protein synthesis in human tenocytes[3]. Human dermal fibroblasts under tension become metabolically very active, producing connective tissue and simultaneously inhibiting matrix degradation[13]. Even 15 minutes of cyclic biaxial mechanical strain applied to human tenocytes results in cellular proliferation[24]. Human tendon fibroblasts experimentally stretched for 15 and 60 min at a frequency of 1 Hz and amplitude of 5% secrete increased amounts of TGF-β, bFGF and PDGF[20]. Application of cyclic load to wounded avian flexor tendons results in epitenon cell migration into the wound[22]. In rabbit patellar tendons, application of a 4% strain provides protection against degradation by bacterial collagenase[19]. Normal tendon movement results in cellular deformation and fluid flow. Experimental application of fluid flow shear stresses to rabbit tenocytes results in upregulation of matrix metalloproteinase I and III, possibly an important mechanism for tendon remodeling or injury[4]. Mechanical loading of cells in monolayer or three dimensional constructs can result in increased cell proliferation and collagen synthesis[5].

The precise mechanism by which cells respond to load remains to be elucidated. However, cells must respond to mechanical and chemical signals in a co-ordinated fashion. Intercellular communication to mount mitogenic and matrigenic responses is achieved via gap junctions ex vivo[6].

Early weight bearing following Achilles tendon rupture

Traditionally, most surgeons in Europe would probably opt for operative management followed by below-the-knee cast immobilization in physically active patients[16]. The cast is applied with the ankle in plantar flexion for 2 weeks, during which patients remain non-weight-bearing. At 2 weeks, the cast is removed, the wound examined, and another non-weight-bearing cast with the ankle in less equinus is applied for a further 2 weeks. At 4 weeks from the operation, the cast is again changed, the ankle is positioned so that the foot is plantigrade, and weight-bearing is begun. The cast is removed at 6 weeks. Good and reliable results have been shown with this regimen[10].

However, this regimen leads to ankle stiffness, muscle hypotrophy and prolonged periods on crutches. Early weight-bearing with the foot plantigrade produced good results after surgical repair of acute Achilles tendon ruptures[18]. A prospective longitudinal study (Grade III evidence) was performed to compare the suggested benefits of early weight bearing compared with traditional non-weight-bearing for 6 weeks[17]. In group 1, patients were allowed to bear weight on the tip toes of the operated leg as tolerated, but they were told to keep the leg elevated as much as possible for the first 2 post-operative weeks[15]. At 2 weeks, the cast was removed for wound check, and a synthetic anterior below-the-knee slab was applied, with the ankle in neutral position. The slab was secured to the leg with three or four removable Velcro straps for 4 weeks. These patients were encouraged to bear weight on the operated limb as soon as they felt comfortable, and to gradually progress to full weight-bearing. The patients were seen by a trained physical therapist who taught them to perform gentle mobilization exercises of the ankle, isometric contraction of the gastrocnemius/soleus muscle complex, and gentle concentric contraction of the calf muscles. Patients were encouraged to perform mobilization of the involved ankle several times per day after unstrapping the two most distal straps. Six weeks after surgery, the anterior slab was removed. Group II had traditional non-weight-bearing casts changed at 2, 4, 6, weeks post-operatively with gradual change in position of ankle from plantigrade to neutral.

Patients in group I discarded their crutches at an average of 2.5 weeks from the operation compared with an average of 5.5 weeks in group II. Group I subjects had fewer outpatient visits, and more patients were satisfied with the results of surgery. There was no significant difference in isometric strength and muscle hypotrophy between the two groups despite early range of motion and weight bearing in group I.

Lansdaal and co-workers reported their results on 163 consecutive Achilles tendon ruptures treated by a minimally invasive surgical technique and functional after-treatment[14]. Their post-operative regimen included mobilization on crutches on the first post-operative day and non-weight bearing on the injured leg for 5 days. Then, the plaster is held in place by a semi-rigid tape, or a soft cast is applied. After 1 week, the patient can start full weight bearing and return every 2 weeks for changing of the soft cast, wound inspection and mobilization instructions. A normal walking pattern and isometric muscle exercises are encouraged from the second post-operative week. Peak stress situations should be avoided during the first 3 months. After 6 weeks, the semi-rigid tape is removed and the patient can continue with the mobilization. The median time for the patients to return to their work was 28 days. The median time for the patients to return to full sports activity was 167 days. Ninety-two per cent of patients were either very satisfied or satisfied. Among complications, there were 4 re-ruptures in 163 patients (2.4%).

A recent meta-analysis (Grade II evidence) by Suchak had found only six prospective randomized controlled trials comparing an early functional protocol with the traditional postoperative protocols in acute Achilles tendon rupture repair[21]. Early functional treatment protocols led to excellent subjective responses compared with postoperative immobilization. The re-rupture rate, superficial and deep infection rates in the early functional treatment group was not different to that in the immobilized group. Complications, including scar adhesions and transient sural nerve deficits, occurred less frequently in the early functional treatment group than in the immobilized group. They recommended larger powered, prospective randomized studies to investigate the individual component of early weight-bearing and early range of motion to determine their effects on the outcome of Achilles tendon rupture repair and lead to dynamic rehabilitation protocols to improve patient satisfaction and clinical outcome.

References

1] Akeson WH, Woo SL, Amiel D, Coutts RD, Daniel D. The connective tissue response to immobility: biochemical changes in periarticular connective tissue of the immobilized rabbit knee. Clinical Orthop 1973;93:356-362.

2] Akeson WH, Amiel D, Mechanic GL, Woo SL, Harwood FL, Hamer ML. Collagen cross-linking alterations in joint contractures: changes in the reducible cross-links in periarticular connective tissue collagen after nine weeks of immobilization. Connect Tissue Res 1977;5:15-19.

3] Almekinders LC, Baynes AJ, Bracey LW. An in vitro investigation into the effects of repetitive motion and nonsteroidal antiinflammatory medication on human tendon fibroblasts. Am J Sports Med
1995;23:119-123.

4] Archambault JM, Elfervig-Wall MK, Tsuzaki M, Herzog W, Banes AJ. Rabbit tendon cells produce
MMP-3 in response to fluid flow without significant calcium transients. J Biomech 2002;35:303-309.

5] Banes AJ, Tsuzaki M, Yamamoto J, Fischer T, Brigman B, Brown T, et al. Mechanoreception at the cellular level: the detection, interpretation, and diversity of responses to mechanical signals. Biochem
Cell Biol 1995;73:349-365.

6] Banes AJ, Horesovsky G, Larson C, Tsuzaki M, Judex S, Archambault J, et al. Mechanical load stimulates expression of novel genes in vivo and in vitro in avian flexor tendon cells. Osteoarth Cartilage
1999;7:141-153.

7] Buckwalter JA. Activity vs. rest in the treatment of bone, soft tissue and joint injuries. Iowa Orthop
J 1995;15:29-42.

8] Buckwalter JA. Effects of early motion on healing of musculoskeletal tissues. Hand Clin 1996;12:13-
24.

9] Chow JA, Thomes LJ, Dovelle S, Monsivais J, Milnor WH, Jackson JP. Controlled motion rehabilitation
after flexor tendon repair and grafting. A multi-centre study. J Bone Joint Surg [Br] 1988;70:591-595.

10] Coutts A, MacGregor A, Gibson J, et al: Clinical and functional results of open operative repair for
Achilles tendon rupture in a non-specialist surgical unit. J R Coll Surg Edinb 2002;47:753–762.

11] Cullen KW, Tolhurst P, Lang D, Page RE. Flexor tendon repair in zone 2 followed by controlled active
mobilisation. Br J Hand Surg 1989;14:392-395.

12] Elliot D, Moiemen NS, Flemming AF, Harris SB, Foster AJ. The rupture rate of acute flexor tendon
repairs mobilized by the controlled active motion regimen. Br J Hand Surg 1994;19:607-612.

13] Kessler D, Dethlefsen S, Haase I, Plomann M, Hirche F, Krieg T, Eckes B. Fibroblasts in mechanically
stressed collagen lattices assume a "synthetic" phenotype. J Biol Chem 2001 28;276:575-585.

14] Lansdaal JR, Goslings JC, Reichart M, Govaert GA, van Scherpenzeel KM, Haverlag R, Ponsen KJ.
The results of 163 Achilles tendon ruptures treated by a minimally invasive surgical technique and
functional aftertreatment. Injury 2007;38:839-844.

15] Maffulli N. Current concepts in the management of subcutaneous tears of the Achilles tendon.
Bull Hosp Jt Dis 1998;57:152–158.

16] Maffulli N: Rupture of the Achilles tendon. J Bone Joint Surg 1999;81A:1019–1036.

17] Maffulli N, Tallon C, Wong J, Lim KP, Bleakney R. Early weightbearing and ankle mobilization after
open repair of acute midsubstance tears of the Achilles tendon. Am J Sports Med.2003;31:692-700.

18] Maffulli N, Tallon C, Wong J, et al: No adverse effect of early weight bearing following open repair
of acute tears of the Achilles tendon. J Sports Med Phys Fit 2003;43:367-379.

19] Nabeshima Y, Grood ES, Sakurai A, Herman JH. Uniaxial tension inhibits tendon collagen degradation by collagenase in vitro. J Orthop Res1996;14:123-130.

20] Skutek M, van Griensven M, Zeichen J, Brauer N, Bosch U. Cyclic mechanical stretching modulates
secretion pattern of growth factors in human tendon fibroblasts. Eur J Appl Physiol 2001;86:48-52.

21] Suchak AA, Spooner C, Reid DC, Jomha NM. Postoperative rehabilitation protocols for Achilles
tendon ruptures: a meta-analysis. Clin Orthop Relat Res 2006;445:216-221.

22] Tanaka H, Manske PR, Pruitt DL, Larson BJ. Effect of cyclic tension on lacerated flexor tendons in
vitro. J Hand Surg Am 1995;20:467-473.

23] Yamamoto E, Hayashi K, Yamamoto N. Mechanical properties of collagen fascicles from stress-
shielded patellar tendons in the rabbit. Clin Biomech1999;14:418-425.

24] Zeichen J, van Griensven M, Bosch U. The proliferative response of isolated human tendon fibroblasts to cyclic biaxial mechanical strain. Am J Sports Med 2000;28:888-892.

*"The greater the obstacle, the
more glory in overcoming it."*

(Molière)

CHAPTER 14.

GUIDELINES FOR SPORT RESUMPTION

Maayke N. van Sterkenburg, Brian G. Donley, C. Niek van Dijk

Take Home Message

• *The time to return to sports after ATR depends on the desired level of sports involvement. The average time before sports can be resumed is 20-24 weeks post-rupture*
• *Patients managed post-operatively using a functional brace can expect to return to their sports on average 4 weeks earlier when compared with patients who received post-operative cast immobilisation*
• *The most important signs which indicate whether it is possible to speed up or it is necessary to slow down the rehabilitation process are pain and swelling after activity as well as delayed tissue healing*

1. Introduction

Traditionally, the most important outcome measures after treatment of an acute rupture of the Achilles tendon have been rerupture, wound complications and infection. Although they are of importance, they can usually be managed. From the patient's point of view, more important outcome measures after an Achilles tendon rupture are the time to return to previous activities such as walking, stair climbing, work, and return to normal sporting activity. In this chapter, we focus on return to sport, which has become an increasingly important outcome measure, probably because of the current keep-fit culture. The average time to return to sports is dependent on which sports the patient practised before the Achilles tendon rupture, and the desired level of sports involvement. For example, return to cycling requires a shorter period of rehabilitation when compared to playing soccer because of the high demands of the game.

In this chapter the physical variables influencing the return to activity and the different levels of activity that can be identified are described, followed by a recommendation concerning the time before different activity levels can be resumed. We based our recommendations on the literature and expert opinions obtained within the Achilles Tendon Study Group.

2. Factors influencing return to activity

Return to preoperative activity level depends mostly on the recovery of different parameters. The tendon needs to be at least partially healed before it can be loaded. It is not only the quality of the healed tendon, that determines whether a patient can resume activities of daily life such as walking and stair climbing or return to sport, however. The range of motion (ROM), especially in dorsiflexion, should be normal to near to normal, and depending on the level of activity, strength and proprioception have to be normalized. Pain and swelling are other factors that might influence a successful return to pre-injury activity level.

2.1 Tissue healing

Tissue healing is the first parameter of importance after an Achilles tendon rupture. In the table below, the different phases of tendon healing following a rupture are described.

Phase			Time
1	Inflammatory phase	Fusion of tendon stumps by a fibrous bridge perpendicular to the rupture. Production of a fibrovascular tendon callus by fibroblast proliferation and type III collagen production.	Weeks 1 and 2
2	Reparative collagen forming phase	Greater orientation along long axis of tendon (as a result of tension being applied on the callus). Increase in the number of intermolecular bonds between collagen fibres increase. Collagen synthesis changes from type III to type I.	Weeks 3 and 4
3	Remodelling phase	Minimal histological difference (vascularity, cellularity) between healed & normal tendon.	Weeks 5 to 20

Table 1: Phases of Achilles tendon rupture healing

Factors affecting recovery in tendon injuries are immobilisation, exercise, age and the possible use of corticosteroids. Immobilised tendons show signs of hypotrophy, collagen fibres become thinner and more disoriented, whereas exercise increases tendon strength[5,6,8,9,16,21,23]. Immobilisation also causes joint stiffness because of the development of synovial adhesions[8,16,23]. In the absence of loading, collagen production decreases and the remodelling to increase the quality of the healing tendon slows down. In older patients, the tendon is stiffer, which affects tendon function[4,5,6,8,9,16,23]. Steroids cause the tendon to become thinner and negatively affect collagen content [16].

2.2. Physical parameters

In addition to tissue healing, other variables might be affected after an Achilles tendon rupture; these include range of motion, proprioception, strength, pain and swelling.

According to the level of activity, a certain degree of recovery on each of these parameters is needed. The patients desired activity level determines the level and quality of recovery that is needed.

3. Activity level

Recovery after an acute rupture of the Achilles tendon can be divided into 4 levels of increasing intensity: walking, running, return to non-contact sports and return to contact sports.
The higher the physical demands, the higher the level and quality of recovery needs to be. Each of these levels of activity demands specific training and exercises. To return to contact sports, the patient first has to achieve the level of normal walking, followed by the level of running and reaching the level of non-contact sports. This demands a systematic expansion of his/her activities, which can be monitored by end terms for each phase. Only when the end terms of each phase are met, the patient can start with specific training in order to optimize speed, force and endurance necessary to progress to the next level. In the following chapter these four levels of activity are further specified.

4. Return to activity

Level 1: The first phase of Achilles tendon rupture healing is return to normal walking. This phase starts at day 0 and ends when the patient is able to walk normally again. The most important factor which determines the return to normal walking is the quality and strength of tissue healing. As the tissue heals, the mechanical properties of the tendon improve, making it possible to increase the load. Patients can switch from unloaded to loaded activity as soon as it is tolerated. After removal of a cast or external support, patients can switch from static to dynamic training. The next step is to proceed from concentric to eccentric muscle training, and, when this is achieved, it will be followed by progression from open to closed chain exercises. Proprioception is trained in order to achieve active stability. An acceptable level of proprioception is reached when the time spent while standing on a single leg is normal or near-normal. ROM should be near normal at the end of phase 1. No passive stretching is allowed in this phase. Concerning strength, there should not be more than a 25% left/right difference which can be measured by performing repeated one leg heel-raises comparing left to right[9]; toe walking should also be possible at this point. Pain and swelling must be absent within 48 hours after increased activity.

When all these variables are similar to those on the unaffected limb, the patient can safely resume unrestricted normal walking without external support.

Level 2: The next level of activity is to resume running. This phase demands recovery of speed, force and endurance. It starts when the patient is able to walk normally and ends when the patient can return to easy jogging. This is achieved by training technical skills, force, endurance and improving the cardiovascular status as well. The goal of this programme is to enable controlled sideward moving and to regain a normal ROM. At the end of this phase there should be a left/right difference in strength of less than 12%. After increased activity, pain and swelling should be absent within 24 hours.

Level 3: The third level of activity is the return to non-contact sports. This involves further training of speed, force and endurance. This phase starts when easy jogging is possible, and ends when the patient is able to return to non-contact sports. It comprises further training of speed to allow running on even ground and sprinting. Muscle strength is equally trained.

At the end of this phase, rope jumping, turning and twisting should be possible, and endurance training is advanced. Muscle strength should be normal, and some pain may occur after increased activity but should be absent after 24 hours.

Level 4: The highest level of activity is defined as the return to contact sports. This phase starts when non-contact sports are resumed, and ends when patients can safely return to contact sports. Final training of speed, muscle strength and endurance should enable the patient to return to contact sports, which involves running on uneven ground, generating explosive force, changing direction and other sports-specific movements.

5. Time to return to sport

There are different factors of importance concerning treatment and rehabilitation, which influence the time and quality of recovery. Based on evidence obtained from the literature and expert opinion, we propose a timeline that can be followed when patients are preparing to return to their preferred sports. The existing literature on return to sport after rupture of the Achilles tendon is summarized below.

5.1. Literature on return to sport in relation to different methods of treating Achilles tendon ruptures

5.1.1. Conservative versus operative treatment

A differentiation can be made in conservatively and surgically-treated patients. Nistor and Moller reported no statistical differences in terms of the reduction of level of sporting activity post-rupture between those 2 groups[18,20]. However, Cetti described that, of 111 patients treated for an acute Achilles tendon rupture, 57% of the surgically-treated group and only 29% of conservatively-treated patients managed to reach the same level of sporting activity as before the injury[2]. Thermann found no difference in functional outcome between surgical and functional-conservative treatment in duration of rehabilitation in a prospective study[22].

5.1.2. Postoperative casting versus functional bracing

Post-operatively, patients may either have a cast or functional bracing.
Maffulli and co-workers reviewed the available concepts on rupture of the Achilles tendon[16]. They found that post-operative functional bracing resulted in a 4 weeks shorter period of return to normal walking compared with post-operative casting, which allowed patients to resume sports 4 weeks earlier. They also felt that post-operative treatment avoiding immobilisation of the ankle should be considered for athletes and well-motivated, reliable patients. At the 4th postoperative week, the ankle should dorsiflect to neutral in a synthetic slab in which plantar flexion is allowed. At 6 weeks, the slab is removed and high-level athletes who comply with the postoperative protocol normally should be able to return to sports activities 12-14 weeks post-operatively.
Costa performed two independent, randomised, controlled trials in order to assess the potential benefits of immediate weight-bearing mobilisation after rupture of the Achilles tendon. The first trial compared post-operative casting to functional bracing. The majority of the patients in both groups had returned to their pre-injury state by six months after the injury[3].
Kangas and co-workers performed a randomised, clinical study from which they concluded that isokinetic calf muscle strength was better in the postoperative functional bracing group. In a second study they investigated subjective outcome measures as pain, stiffness and footwear restrictions and showed similar results for both groups[7]. Mortensen described a period of rehabilitation of 7.5 months in the cast group, compared with 4 months in the functional brace group[19]. Kerkhoffs reported the time to return to sports of 73 days (range 54-112) for a cast group and 57 days (49-70) for a functional brace group[10].
Mortensen also studied the time to reach pre-injury level of activity, and concluded that the functional brace group needed 6 months of recovery compared with 9 months in the cast group[19].

5.1.3. Functional conservative treatment versus plaster cast immobilisation

Costa compared conservative treatment with immediate weight-bearing mobilisation to plaster-cast immobilisation. There was, however, no evidence of a treatment effect in terms of time to return to sports[3].

5.1.4. Percutaneous versus open operative treatment

Lim compared a small group of active patients, who were treated with percutaneous suture to open surgery and noted that 4/9 of the open group reached their pre-injury level of sporting activity compared with 9/11 in the percutaneous group[14]. Lansdaal found that in 163 patients treated with minimally invasive surgery, the average time to return to full sports activity was 167 days[13].

5.2. Proposed time for return to sport

On the basis of the findings described above we came to the following timeline:

Level 1: return to normal walking: The most important factor, which determines the return to normal loading, is the quality of tissue healing. In case of cast immobilisation after surgery, one can expect this phase to last up to 12 weeks. At the end of this 12 week period, the patient should have progressed to unrestricted walking without external support (Level I evidence). In case of functional treatment after surgery, this period is expected to be reduced to 8 weeks[16]. (level III evidence).
Level 2: Recovery of force, speed and endurance: The expert panel recommends this phase to take a minimum of 4-6 weeks (Level V evidence).
Level 3: Return to non-contact sports: This phase can be expected to take another 4-6 weeks (Level V evidence).
Level 4: Return to contact sports: if patients take part in contact sports, this typically needs another 4-6 weeks of rehabilitation. (Level V evidence)

OPERATIVE TREATMENT FOLLOWED BY CAST IMMOBILISATION

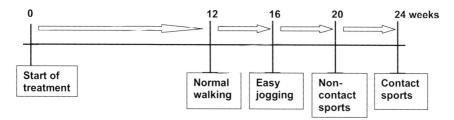

OPERATIVE TREATMENT FOLLOWED BY FUNCTIONAL BRACING

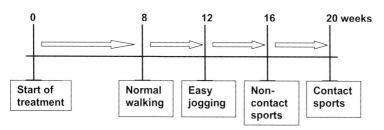

CONSERVATIVE TREATMENT IN CAST OR FUNCTIONAL BRACE

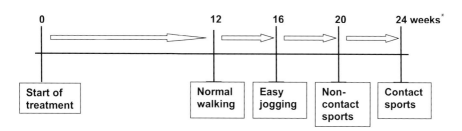

*There is no evidence for a prolonged period of time before sports can be resumed in conservatively treated patients, but a significantly smaller amount of patients is able to return to their previous level of activity [2,18,20,22].

The expected time given to resume each of the activity levels is an average. There are individual differences where one patient is quicker, while another needs more time to reach the same rehabilitation goal. The most important signs to monitor if a patient can speed up or has to slow down on the average time are pain and swelling after activity and delayed tissue healing.

6. Conclusion

The period of time before sporting activities can be resumed after an Achilles tendon rupture depends on a combination of several factors. A well-motivated, compliant athlete can resume sports earlier than someone who is not. Patients who are treated with surgery and post-operative treatment using a functional brace will be able to resume their activities significantly earlier than a conservatively treated patient immobilized in a cast. Also, the time to return to pre-injury level of activity is expected to be shorter in the first group.

RETURN TO SPORT AFTER ACUTE ACHILLES TENDON RUPTURE

PHASE	GOAL	TRAINING OF	DURATION	END TERMS	SPORTS
1: **Tissue Healing**	Return to normal loading	Proprioception	12 weeks[1]	Active Stability (A negative Rhomberg test by standing on one leg)	
		Improve ROM		ROM near normal No passive stretching is allowed	
		Static ⟷ dynamic Eccentric ⟷ Concentric Open Chain ⟷ Closed Chain		Improved Speed, number of repetitions and length of rest period Force < 25% L/R difference measured by performing heel raise test comparing ability of left to right	
				Pain/Swelling after increased activity should be gone < 48 hrs	
					Normal walking
2A: **Recovery of** **Speed, Force &** **Endurance**	Return to Sport Specific Loading	Technical skills	**4 weeks**	Controlled sideward Movements ROM normal	
		Force		Force < 12% L/R difference	
		Endurance Cardiovascular status		Some Pain/Swelling after increased activity should be gone < 24 hrs	
					Easy Jogging

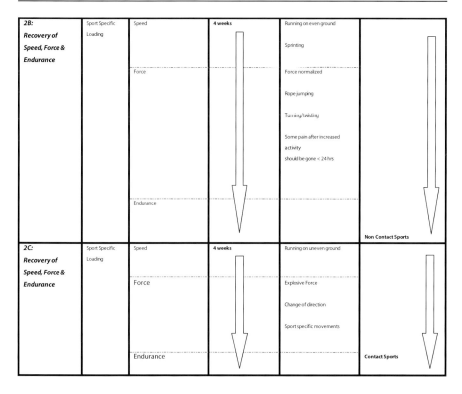

2B: *Recovery of Speed, Force & Endurance*	Sport Specific Loading	Speed	4 weeks	Running on even ground	
				Sprinting	
		Force		Force normalized	
				Rope jumping	
				Turning/twisting	
				Some pain after increased activity should be gone < 24 hrs	
		Endurance			**Non Contact Sports**
2C: *Recovery of Speed, Force & Endurance*	Sport Specific Loading	Speed	4 weeks	Running on uneven ground	
		Force		Explosive Force	
				Change of direction	
				Sport specific movements	
		Endurance			**Contact Sports**

[1] In case of functional bracing after operative treatment for acute Achilles tendon rupture this phase can be shortened to 8 weeks.

Acknowledgement

The financial support of the Stichting amphoraest (Foundation) is acknowledged.

Reference List

1] Akizuki KH, Gartman EJ, Nisonson B, Ben-Avi S, McHugh MP. The relative stress on the Achilles tendon during ambulation in an ankle immobiliser: implications for rehabilitation after Achilles tendon repair. Br J Sports Med 2001;35:329-333.

2] Cetti R, Christensen SE, Ejsted R, Jensen NM, Jorgensen U. Operative versus nonoperative treatment of Achilles tendon rupture. A prospective randomized study and review of the literature. Am J Sports Med 1993;21:791-799.

3] Costa ML, MacMillan K, Halliday D, Chester R, Shepstone L, Robinson AH, et al. Randomised controlled trials of immediate weight-bearing mobilisation for rupture of the tendo Achillis. J Bone Joint Surg Br 2006;88:69-77.

4] Evans NA, Stanish WD. The basic science of tendon injuries. Curr Orthop 2000;14: 403-412.

5] Järvinen M, Jozsa L, Kannus P, Järvinen TL, Kvist M, Leadbetter W. Histopathological findings in chronic tendon disorders. Scand J Med Sci Sports 1997;7:86-95.

6] Jozsa L, Kannus P. Histopathological findings in spontaneous tendon ruptures. Scand J Med Sci Sports 1997;7:113-118.

7] Kangas J, Pajala A, Siira P, Hamalainen M, Leppilahti J. Early functional treatment versus early immobilization in tension of the musculotendinous unit after Achilles rupture repair: a prospective, randomized, clinical study. J Trauma 2003;54:1171-1180.

8] Kannus P, Jozsa L, Natri A, Jarvinen M. Effects of training, immobilization and remobilization on tendons. Scand J Med Sci Sports 1997;7:67-71.

9] Kannus P, Natri A. Etiology and pathophysiology of tendon ruptures in sports. Scand J Med Sci Sports 1997;7:107-112.

10] Kerkhoffs GM, Struijs PA, Raaymakers EL, Marti RK. Functional treatment after surgical repair of acute Achilles tendon rupture: wrap vs walking cast. Arch Orthop Trauma Surg 2002;122:102-105.

11] Khan RJ, Fick D, Keogh A, Crawford J, Brammar T, Parker M. Treatment of acute achilles tendon ruptures. A meta-analysis of randomized, controlled trials. J Bone Joint Surg Am 2005;87:2202-2210.

12] Kocher MS, Bishop J, Marshall R, Briggs KK, Hawkins RJ. Operative versus nonoperative management of acute Achilles tendon rupture: expected-value decision analysis. Am J Sports Med 2002;30:783-790.

13] Lansdaal JR, Goslings JC, Reichart M, Govaert GA, van Scherpenzeel KM, Haverlag R, et al. The results of 163 Achilles tendon ruptures treated by a minimally invasive surgical technique and functional aftertreatment. Injury 2007;38:839-844.

14] Lim J, Dalal R, Waseem M. Percutaneous vs. open repair of the ruptured Achilles tendon--a prospective randomized controlled study. Foot Ankle Int 2001;22:559-568.

15] Lunsford BR, Perry J. The standing heel-rise test for ankle plantar flexion: criterion for normal. Phys Ther 1995;75:694-698.

16] Maffulli N. Rupture of the Achilles tendon. J Bone Joint Surg Am 1999;81:1019-1036.

17] McComis GP, Nawoczenski DA, DeHaven KE. Functional bracing for rupture of the Achilles tendon. Clinical results and analysis of ground-reaction forces and temporal data. J Bone Joint Surg Am 1997;79:1799-1808.

18] Möller M, Movin T, Granhed H, Lind K, Faxén E, Karlsson J. Acute rupture of tendon Achillis. A prospective randomised study of comparison between surgical and non-surgical treatment. J Bone Joint Surg Br 2001;83:843-848.

19] Mortensen HM, Skov O, Jensen PE. Early motion of the ankle after operative treatment of a rupture of the Achilles tendon. A prospective, randomized clinical and radiographic study. J Bone Joint Surg Am 1999;81:983-990.

20] Nistor L. Surgical and non-surgical treatment of Achilles tendon rupture. J Bone Joint Surg 1981;63:394-399.

21] Novacheck TF. Running injuries: a biomechanical approach. Instr Course Lect 1998;47:397-406.

22] Thermann H, Zwipp H, Tscherne H. [Functional treatment concept of acute rupture of the Achilles tendon. 2 years results of a prospective randomized study]. Unfallchirurg 1995;98:21-32.

23] Woo SL, Gelberman RH, Cobb NG, Amiel D, Lothringer K, Akeson WH. The importance of controlled passive mobilization on flexor tendon healing. A biomechanical study. Acta Orthop Scand 1981;52:615-622.

CHAPTER 15.

OUTCOME MEASURES AND SCORING SYSTEMS

Aimee C. Stroink, Karin Grävare Silbernagel, Jon Karlsson, C. Niek van Dijk

Take Home Message

• *For evaluating outcome after treatment of acute Achilles tendon rupture it is important to use reliable, valid and sensitive outcome measures.*
• *It is also important to not only use one outcome measure since the aspects of patients' satisfaction and function are multifactorial.*
• *We therefore recommend the use of both patient-reported questionnaires along with various tests of function.*

Introduction

Evidence based medicine is widely accepted and for evaluating and comparing research studies, valid and reliable outcome measures are needed. Such assessment parameters can also be used as guidelines for prognosis and assist physicians and patients in the decision-
making process. In recent years, the demand for validated, reliable and responsive outcome measures which are injury-specific has been growing. An overview of outcome measures and scoring systems concerning the acute Achilles tendon ruptures will be given in this chapter.
Previously scoring systems that combined both subjective and objective param-

eters have been used. The Hannover Achilles tendon score as the modified score of Boyden is one such system, however, it is hard to appraise, since it combines scoring systems, which aggregate subjective (patient satisfaction) and objective (clinician-assessed measures) findings.

In this chapter, the aim is to review outcome measures, which are usable in both research and clinical settings, evaluating symptoms, physical parameters, strength and function. Their use, the documented validity and reliability for evaluating outcome after Achilles tendon rupture will also be reported.

Outcome measures and scoring systems

When comparing the outcome of treatments following Achilles tendon rupture, it is often the risk of complications such as reruptures, infections, adhesions and disturbed skin sensibility, which are being compared. The complications are usually reported in terms of relative risk or percentage. Furthermore, comparisons in regards to length of hospital stay, time off work and return to sports are often made. This type of documentation does not require any specific tools; however, it requires that all patients in a research study will be followed over time and that these aspects are reported in a standardized way in order to perform future comparisons between different research studies. Another chapter of this current concepts book will discuss the aspect of return to sports more thoroughly.

Patients' satisfaction along with objective assessments of, for example strength, endurance and range of motion are also of utmost importance when comparing various treatment options. Almost all traditional parameters, after treatment of Achilles tendon pathology, like pain, limp range of motion, calf circumference, isokinetic strength measurements, have not been convincingly correlated with clinical outcome and patient satisfaction[4,5,6]. It can therefore be recommended to use several different types of outcome measures in order to establish a complete picture of the outcome of treatment following acute Achilles tendon rupture.

Questionnaires

The Achilles Tendon Total Rupture Score - ATRS

Until recently, there has not been any injury-specific questionnaire available for evaluating outcome after treatment for acute Achilles tendon rupture. In 2007, Nilsson-Helander and co-workers developed a patient-reported instrument for evaluating outcome in patients with total Achilles tendon rupture[13]. The ATRS evaluates aspects of symptoms and physical activity. The questionnaire consists of 10 items, where the score for each item ranges between 0-10 on a Likert scale, with a maximal score of 100. The total score for patients in their study ranged from 17 to 100 with a mean of 77 (SD 21.4). A significantly (p<.0001) higher total score was found for the healthy subjects ranging from 94 to 100 with a mean of 99.8 (SD 1.1). The questionnaire was further evaluated and was shown to have good reliability, validity and responsiveness for evaluating outcome after treatment in patients with Acute Achilles tendon rupture (Table 1). The patients can complete the questionnaire in a couple of minutes and it is easy for the clinician to score.

In summary, this questionnaire can be recommended to be used both in research and every day clinical work.

The American Orthopaedic Foot and Ankle Society clinical rating system - AOFAS

The American Orthopaedic Foot and Ankle Society (AOFAS) has developed four rating systems, in which the clinical status of the ankle and foot is reported[8]. The purpose of these rating systems was to have a clinically useful method, which could be used when comparing the results of different methods of treatment. These systems incorporate both subjective and objective factors. The AOFAS Ankle-Hindfoot scale may seem appropriate to use to evaluate patient-related outcome after Achilles tendon rupture, however, it is described to be used for ankle replacement, ankle arthrodesis, ankle instability operations, subtalar arthrodesis, subtalar instability operations, talo-navicular arthrodesis, calcaneo-cuboid arthrodesis, calcaneal osteotomy, calcaneus fracture, talus fracture and ankle fracture[8]. These types of injuries are very different from Achilles tendon ruptures and the symptoms and factors affecting outcome are not similar. Such ratings as pain and hindfoot motion and ankle-hindfoot stability appear to have low face validity for patients with Achilles tendon ruptures. Even though the AOFAS ankle-hindfoot scale has been used as outcome measure in studies on Achilles tendon rupture it cannot be recommended since it has not been evaluated for reliability, validity and responsiveness in this patient population.

The Foot and Ankle Outcome Score - FAOS

The Foot and Ankle Outcome Score[17] is another patient-reported questionnaire which evaluates symptoms and functional limitations related to the foot and ankle. It assess five different dimensions such as pain, other symptoms (stiffness, swelling and range of motion), activities of daily living, sports and recreational activities and foot and ankle related quality of life. FAOS has been evaluated for reliability and validity in patients with ankle ligament reconstruction. It has, however, not been evaluated in patients with acute Achilles tendon rupture. Several questions in FAOS appears to have low face validity for evaluating patients with Achilles tendon ruptures and is more time consuming, which makes its clinical utility less in comparison with the ATRS. However, certain parts of the FAOS, such as quality of life section may be useful in evaluating other aspects of patient satisfaction with treatment. This questionnaire might therefore be a good addition to the ATRS in both the clinic and research.

Patient reported classification systems - Questionnaires		
Achilles tendon total rupture score **ATRS**	Validated: yes Test-retest reliability: ICC 0.98 Internal consistency (Cronbach's alpha) 0.96 Correlation with (subscales) of VISA-A-S (r=0.78) FAOS (r=0.60-0.84) Responsiveness 0.87-2.21	The ATRS is a self-administered instrument with high clinical utility. It can be recommended to be used in both research and in the clinical setting.
The American Orthopaedic Foot and Ankle Society clinical rating system - **AOFAS**	Not evaluated on patients with acute Achilles tendon ruptures	These systems incorporate both subjective and objective factors. Parts of the rating system appear to have low face validity. Needs to be evaluated on patients with Achilles tendon rupture prior to being recommended for use.
Foot and Ankle Outcome Score **FAOS**	Shown to have good reliability and validity in patients with ankle ligament reconstruction Not evaluated on patients with acute Achilles tendon ruptures	Evaluates various dimensions, which are not evaluated by the ATRS and could therefore be used along with the ATRS. However it needs to be further evaluated on patients with acute Achilles tendon rupture.

Table 1: Summary of patient-reported outcome measures

Physical exam measurements

Calf circumference/muscle atrophy

Circumference measurements are often used clinically to determine gross muscular hypotrophy; however, such measurements can not be used to determine muscle quality. Techniques include documenting maximum circumference or measuring at predetermined positions relating to bony landmarks[15]. Möller and co-workers found good reliability for calf circumference measurements (ICC 0.97)[12]. It is important to remember that circumference measurements are affected by swelling and body composition (fat versus muscle) and increases in circumference may not indicate increased muscle mass or vice versa. Furthermore, the calf muscle circumference has a weak correlation to calf muscle strength and endurance after treatment for Achilles tendon rupture[11]. However, when calf muscle cross-sectional area is derived from CT scans it correlates well with the muscle's working capacity measured as the number of heel raises. To summarize, calf circumference might be a tool to be used in the clinic, however, it can not be recommended for use in research as a measure relating to function. In research measures derived from CT scans might instead be of use.

Ankle range of motion

Measurements of range of motion are usually performed in the clinic and also in research studies. Since one complication of acute Achilles tendon rupture is tendon elongation, the range of motion measure can be used as an indirect measure of tendon elongation. In other words, increased dorsiflexion is assumed to be associated with Achilles tendon elongation. Goniometric measurements can be performed in the supine or standing positions and both actively and passively while maintaining the foot in a subtalar neutral position. The arms of the goniometer should be aligned, with the proximal arm along the midline of the fibula, the fulcrum by the lateral malleoli and the distal arm parallel to the fifth metatarsal[14]. Regular goniometric range of motion evaluations have been shown to be reliable, with intra-tester reliability being higher than inter-tester reliability[3,18]. Range of motion measurements of the ankle have been used in several research studies as an outcome measures when evaluating various treatments.

Strength test

The reliability of isokinetic and isometric dynamometry is generally high and the various testing positions of plantarflexion and dorsiflexion have shown good test-retest reliability[1,12]. The results from isokinetic testing can be influenced by the test procedure and this therefore should be thoroughly documented in research studies. Strength tests are valid for measuring improvements in strength, but they are moderately correlated to functional performance and are hard to perform in every clinical setting due to the expensive and large equipment. It is therefore recommended to complement strength measurements with dynamometry with other types of functional assessment.

Endurance test

Muscular endurance testing is another type of muscle function measurement. In a heel rise test (also called toe-raise or heel-drop), the plantarflexion of the ankle is performed repetitively while standing until fatigued. It is the most commonly used test for measuring the muscular endurance of the calf musculature. The normal number of toe-raise repetitions on one leg is regarded to be approximately 25, but it can range from six to 70 in healthy individuals[9]. The testing position for the subject is standing on one leg while maintaining a straight knee, support with the fingertips for balance and avoiding body sway forward. Häggmark and co-workers also used a light beam at a height of five cm above the floor and only the number of heel rises above the light beam was counted[5]. This test has been used in several research studies and has shown good reliability (ICC 0.78-0.84)[20,21,12].

A correlation between isokinetic strength measurement and the heel rise test was reported by Möller and co-workers[11]. Since the heel-rise test is clinical more practicable it can recommended for measuring the calf muscle function in both research and clinic.

Imaging methods

Concerning the radiographic scoring systems; no consistence is found between the correlation on ultrasonographic changes and the clinical outcome measures. Rupp and co-workers[19] as well as Möller and co-workers[11] found no correlation between the findings, whereas Rominger and co-workers[16] showed a positive correlation with general symptoms and (p<0.001), pain on movement (p<0.001), reduced function (p=0.005), and reduced sporting activity (p=0.034).

These different results can be caused due to the different outcome measures used by the authors. In contrast to Rominger and co-workers[16] who had splitted all their findings, Rupp and co-workers[19] used their own, non-validated outcome measure, which consisted of subjective, as well as objective measurements.

Rominger and co-workers[16] also found a positive and significant correlation between ultrasound and MR imaging for morphometric and morphological changes (p<0.001. p=0.004). This reproducibility of the US and MR imaging evaluation was confirmed for the sagittal dimension by Möller and co-workers[11].

All investigated authors[2,10,11,19] found greater antero-posterior diameter of the ruptured tendon, but only Bleakney and co-workers[2] as well as Maffulli and co-workers[10] mentioned that this difference was of a significant order.

The consensus is that radiodiagnostic studies play a limited role during the healing period of patients treated for Achilles tendon rupture.

When evaluating the results of objective findings, for patients who sustained an Achilles tendon rupture, restraint should be obtained with interpreting the results. An abnormal image or measurement does not necessarily imply poor function or clinical relevant pathology.

As quoted by Khan and co-workers in 1998[7]: "Treat the patient not the X-ray".

Physical exam measurements		
Calf circumference	Reliability: ICC 0.97 0.98 Validity: Questionable	Easily used in the clinic Weak correlation to calf muscle strength and endurance.
Ankle range of motion Goniometric evaluation	Reliability: ICC 0.71-0.91 Validity: High for measuring ROM Not evaluated for measuring tendon elongation	Easily used in the clinic and research. May be a clinical tool for determining tendon elongation.
Isokinetic testing (different positions)	Reliability: Plantarflexion ICC 0.53-0.95 Dorsiflexion ICC 0.00-0.95 Valid for measuring strength	Good for measuring strength but moderately correlated with function. Usable in clinic and research
Heel-raise test for endurance	Reliability: ICC 0.78-0.84 Valid for measuring endurance of the calf musculature	Good clinical utility and usable in research.
Radiographic scoring systems	No correlation between ultrasonographic changes and clinical outcome measures.	Radiodiagnostic imaging play a limited role during the healing period of patients treated for Achilles tendon rupture

Table 2: Summary of the physical examination outcome measures

References

1] Alfredson H, Pietilä T, Öhberg L, Lorentzon R. Achilles tendinosis and calf muscle strength. The effect of short-term immobilization after surgical treatment. Am J Sports Med 1998;26:166-171.

2] Bleakney RR, White LM. Imaging of the Achilles tendon. Foot Ankle Clin 2005;10:239-254.

3] Boone DC, Azen SP, Lin CM, Spence C, Baron C, Lee L. Reliability of goniometric measurements. Phys Ther 1978;58:1355-1390.

4] Cetti R et al. Operative versus nonoperative treatment of Achilles tendon rupture. A prospective randomized study and review of the literature. Am J Sports Med 1993;21:791-799.

5] Häggmark T, Eriksson E. Hypotrophy of the soleus muscle in man after achilles tendon rupture. Discussion of findings obtained by computed tomography and morphologic studies. Am J Sports Med 1979;7:121-126.

6] Häggmark T et al. Calf muscle atrophy and muscle function after non-operative vs operative treatment of achilles tendon ruptures. Orthopedics 1986;9:160-164.

7] Khan KM et al. Treat the patient, not the x-ray: advances in diagnostic imaging do not replace the need for clinical interpretation. Clin J Sport Med 1998;8:1-4.

8] Kitaoka HB, Alexander IJ, Adelaar RS, Nunley JA, Myerson MS, Sanders M. Clinical rating systems for the ankle-hindfoot, midfoot, hallux, and lesser toes. Foot Ankle Int 1994;15:349-353.

9] Lunsford BR, Perry J. The standing heel-rise test for ankle plantar flexion: criterion for normal. Phys Ther 1995;75:694-698.

10] Maffulli N, Thorpe AP, and Smith FW. Magnetic resonance imaging after operative repair of Achilles tendon rupture. Scandinavian Journal of Medicine & Science in Sports 2001;11:156-162.

11] Möller M et al. The ultrasonographic appearance of the ruptured Achilles tendon during healing: a longitudinal evaluation of surgical and nonsurgical treatment, with comparisons to MRI appearance. Knee Surg Sports Traumatol Arthrosc 2002;10: 49-56.

12] Möller M et al. The reliability of isokinetic testing of the ankle joint and a heel-raise test for endurance. Knee Surg Sports Traumatol Arthrosc 2005;13:60-71.

13] Nilsson-Helander K et al. The Achilles Tendon Total Rupture Score (ATRS): Development and Validation. Am J Sports Med 2007.

14] Norkin CC, White DJ. Measurement of joint motion: a guide to goniometry. Philadelphia: Davis; 1985.

15] Paavola M, Kannus P, Orava S, Pasanen M, Järvinen M. Surgical treatment for chronic Achilles tendinopathy: a prospective seven month follow up study. Br J Sports Med 2002;36:178-182.

16] Rominger MB et al. The value of ultrasound and MRI following surgical treatment of rupture of the Achilles tendon. Rofo-Fortschritte Auf dem Gebiet der Rontgenstrahlen und der Bildgebenden Verfahren 1998;168:27-35.

17] Roos EM, Brandsson S, and Karlsson J. Validation of the foot and ankle outcome score for ankle ligament reconstruction. Foot & Ankle International 2001;22:788-794.

18] Rothstein JM, Miller PJ, Roettger RF. Goniometric reliability in a clinical setting. Elbow and knee measurements Phys Ther 1983;63:1611-1615.

19] Rupp S, Tempelhof S, and Fritsch E. Ultrasound of the Achilles-Tendon After Surgical Repair - Morphology and Function. British Journal of Radiology 1995;68:454-458.

20] Svantesson U, Osterberg U, Thomee R, Peeters M, Grimby G. Fatigue during repeated eccentric-concentric and pure concentric muscle actions of the plantar flexors. Clin Biomech (Bristol, Avon)1998;13:336-343.

21] Svantesson U, Österberg U, Thomeé R, Grimby G. Muscle fatigue in a standing heel-rise test. Scand J Rehabil Med 1998;30:67-72.